I'm so happy that Larry has written *The Urb...* myself, I see firsthand the wellness moveme... how the standard Western medical "health ... *Body Fix* advocates and promotes true wellness, as Larry calls it "vibrant health." This book will be a valuable tool for anyone looking to keep themselves and their families in true health. Larry is a rare breed of health care professional who believes in the middle ground. You will never hear Larry advocating for any fad diet or extreme detox. I'm blessed to know Larry and get to hear his pearls of wisdom on a one-to-one basis. Larry's voice comes through clearly and accurately in *The Urban Body Fix*. Now people all over the world can experience his wisdom.

Thank you, Larry for writing this book. I look forward to referring it to all my clients who are on their wellness journeys.

ALYSE FAITH SHYNE, LMT, OWNER AND FOUNDER, THE HEALING COLLECTIVE NY

Larry Rogowsky and *The Urban Body Fix* have accomplished a rare feat in this book: that of delivering a broad range of unique wellness including mental, physical, theoretical and practical tips with a conscious voice that stem from his own depth of experience. Expect the unexpected when reading this gem. If a naturopathic doctor/ epidemiologist with more than 20 years of experience in the integrative medicine space can learn and be inspired at the seeming ease with which this information was joyfully shared, I trust you will be hooked on Larry's style of health coaching. Pick it up today!

DR. MILLIE LYTLE ND, MPH, FOUNDER OF WWW.NATMEDCOACH.COM

The Urban Body Fix is full of wonderful and practical strategies for so many health-related challenges that people are experiencing every day. It's truly a detailed list of all of the best alternative healthcare and wellness tools for so many health problems or struggles many people have. The wisdom Larry shares from years of experience will help so many navigate successfully through many common health challenges, and do it in a safe and natural way. This book is an excellent resource that every human on this planet should read!

KATE MOTZ, NATIONAL BOARD CERTIFIED FUNCTIONAL MEDICINE COACH, FOUNDER OF INTEGRATIVE WELLNESS ADVISORS

Larry does a great job at stating the problem, any barriers that you might potentially face and provides tangible ways (leaving no room for excuses) to live a healthier life on your terms versus the status quo. It touches on ancient, alternative methods to healing the body which gives readers who might not be familiar, new ways of addressing their well-being. This is not a diet book; better it is a comprehensive read, great for anyone starting or needing to redefine their health on their terms.

JENNIFER JONES, OWNER AND FOUNDER OF JENUINE NUTRITION

As I read *The Urban Body Fix*, I was amazed how much I already knew from listening to Larry as his client for the past 15 years. My health has only been getting better as I age, and that is thanks to Larry's wisdom and sensible, doable approach to taking care of my body and mind. The Urban Body Fix comprises all the gentle and supportive reminders I need to keep in vibrant health. Thank you Larry for your inspiring and actionable book. Highly recommended.

BOAZ GILAD, FOUNDER OF AMAST.COM, BUSINESS OWNER, AUTHOR OF *THE REAL ESTATE MILLIONAIRE*

Today, we are looking at a great divide with a leadership gap, and I am not speaking politics here. I am referring to the polarized Wellness paradigm, where on one hand sitting on the couch, binge-watching Netflix has become a celebrated self-care activity and on the other hand, the amazing transformation pictures of fit Instagram models have become a dime a dozen. For the rest of us, we need new leadership. Larry Rogowsky, in his new book *The Urban Body Fix*, presents a no-nonsense, science-based, balanced, and relevant approach to Wellness. Find practical tips such as the benefit of a health-oriented goal (vs. a physique goal), ways to get laughter in (a necessity for your health), and the idea of a "fitness snack" (it's not what you think). Kudos to the presentation of the chapters on Supplements and the Heart-Gut Axis which contain plenty of insider health information. *The Urban Body Fix* will help you attain moderation, so you can live an extraordinary life.

DR. PATRICIA PIMENTEL SELASSIE, NATUROPATHIC DOCTOR, AUTHOR OF *AGING BRILLIANTLY*, DOCTORSELASSIE.COM

I recommend Larry but I married him so what choice do I have?

DREW GERACI, ROGOWSKY FAMILY STAFF

THE
URBAN
BODY FIX

THE
URBAN BODY FIX

EVERYTHING IN MODERATION
(ESPECIALLY MODERATION)

LARRY ROGOWSKY
WITH LOU DONATO

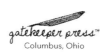

gatekeeper press™
Columbus, Ohio

The Urban Body Fix:
Everything In Moderation (Especially Moderation)

Published by Gatekeeper Press
2167 Stringtown Rd, Suite 109
Columbus, OH 43123-2989
www.GatekeeperPress.com

Copyright © 2021 by Larry Rogowsky and Lou Donato

All rights reserved. Neither this book, nor any parts within it may be sold or reproduced in any form or by any electronic or mechanical means, including information storage and retrieval systems without permission in writing from the author. The only exception is by a reviewer, who may quote short excerpts in a review.

The cover design, interior formatting, typesetting, and editorial work for this book are entirely the product of the author. Gatekeeper Press did not participate in and is not responsible for any aspect of these elements.

ISBN (paperback): 9781662908828
eISBN: 9781662908835

WITH THANKS

To Dad,
who did yoga before it was fashionable

To Mom,
whose care as a nurse reflected her love to everyone

To Drew,
for being my guinea pig when it comes to all things wellness

To Anthony,
the next brave generation of what's possible with excellent health choices

To Sue G.,
who never gave up on me and this book

Table of Contents

Foreword

with Tony Award Winning Actress Stephanie J. Block

———

I have been the beneficiary of Larry Rogowsky's care for many years. Our relationship began based on a recommendation for massage therapy and body work. As a Broadway actress, dedicating my life to a career of performing 8 shows a week, well, it can wreak havoc on the body, the mind and the immune system. Being recommended to spend my day(s) off "under the hands" of Larry was a true gift. It was clear very early on that Larry's skills, knowledge, love of life and people were infused with how he treated both the body and the soul of his clients.

As I read *The Urban Body Fix*, I smiled with great pride and comfort in recognizing that his care translated onto each page. You can feel his investment...his investment toward the search for holistic health and a higher consciousness. He's invested in you, in his fellow person searching to live a vibrant way of life. He writes from example, to this I can attest. He is vibrant as a husband, a father, a healer, a producer and now an author and teacher. And now **YOU** will be the beneficiary of his passion and knowledge. You are able to receive the gift of *The Urban Body Fix*.

This incredible book of awareness, of paying attention to what makes one whole and vibrant couldn't have come at a better time. We are all living in an age where the meter of our lives is on a constant loop of uncertainty, of worry, of deadlines, of disappointment, of pure exhaustion. We are living during a time of divide, a time where we question what is truth and what is simply noise. Amongst all of these detrimental preoccupations, we can lose what makes us feel joyful and purposeful and peaceful...what makes us feel fully alive.

The Urban Body Fix will act as a reset. This book will lead you to what feels right to/for you. It will engage you to want to invest in yourself so that amongst all of the aforementioned distractions, you can always return to what you know your mind, body and spirit responds to. It is only through recognizing what works for you and what doesn't that you are in control of your "whole health", otherwise you will be controlled by imbalance and the latest fad, neither of which will serve you well. I have gone down both roads, the road of extreme and the road of temporary fixes. Both roads will lead to a path of lacking. I am reminded of the saying "Just because you can, doesn't mean you should". Thank goodness at my age, that lesson has been learned. But the lesson of balance and consistency is a daily lesson. That is why I will be using this book as a guide, a reminder and a reference.

I pride myself on living truthfully and joyfully and now, with the help of Larry (once again) I am going to renew my life of vibrancy.

Happy reading and congratulations on investing in your whole health.

Much joy,
Stephanie J. Block

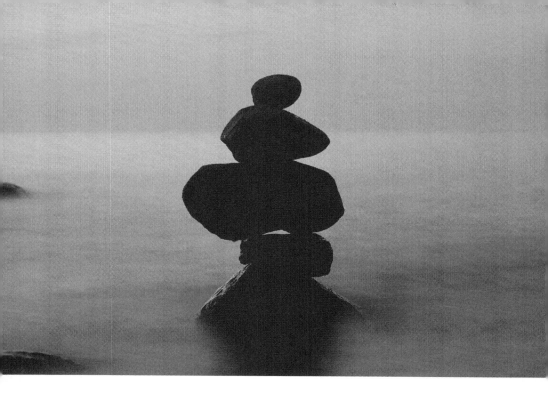

CHAPTER 01

Living Fully by Practicing Moderation in All Things

(Especially Moderation)

Ours is a culture of excess and extreme. There's no better illustration of that than what we do with (*and to!*) our bodies, often in the name of health and fitness, or at least what we've come to perceive those concepts to be. With each generation, Americans find new ways of pushing the boundaries of what humans can and should do, while ignoring blaring indicators that something isn't quite right.

- The list of eating disorders that was once limited to anorexia and bulimia now includes orthorexia and bigorexia and is no longer just a female issue.

- We don't just cut calories anymore, we eliminate entire food groups. We still get breast augmentation, but we also get butt implants.

- A 26.2 mile marathon is too short and too conventional, so now we've got ultramarathons and Death Races.

- Silicon Valley tech executives brag of going days without food and running on two hours of sleep.

- Even our television viewing habits have become more extreme. A single episode of a program is no longer enough so we binge-watch the entire series...on a 75-inch screen, while eating a party-size bag of chips and slurping a 42-ounce "supersized" soft drink.

So how did we get here? How did we become what Columbia University professor Jeffrey Sachs refers to as a "mass-addiction society"?

THE PSYCHOLOGY OF EXTREME

We know that rates of anxiety and depression have gone up considerably in recent years. We're more stressed about life and more unhappy with ourselves. A study out of the University of Texas at Austin determined that binge-eating and binge-watching are associated with depression, loneliness, deficiency, and obesity.

Pleasurable activities like those described above trigger the release of dopamine, the body's "happy hormone." Our brain remembers that feeling and, naturally, we crave more of it. It's not unlike what happens to the body with drug addiction. Any addiction will lead to tolerance, a situation in which we require increasing doses of that pleasurable experience to achieve the same level of happiness we did the previous time. Once we're hooked, other activities are no longer as interesting to us and become less and less of a priority.

The theory of hedonic adaptation helps to explain some of these human tendencies. According to psychologists, the more we experience pleasure, the more we come to expect it. A new activity that is exciting initially soon becomes routine. The happiness is short-lived. Once it fades, it drops back down to baseline level. At this point, we need to aim higher to achieve happiness once again. This phenomenon has been called the "hedonic treadmill" and refers to the perpetual chase of increasingly lofty aspirations just to feel content.

As with drugs, addiction to extreme diet and exercise protocols typically stem from underlying emotional issues. Once upon a time, it was the magazine industry defining and reinforcing the "thin-ideal," the slender female figure by which all others should be judged. Soon after, popular television programs began depicting heavier women in unflattering and disparaging ways. The image of an underweight female became internalized and surveys would show that a majority of women were unhappy with their bodies.

Cases of eating disorders increased dramatically during the late 1970s and early 1980s. Karen Carpenter's death in 1983 led to an increased awareness of anorexia. In 1987, the American Psychiatric Association listed bulimia as its own disorder for the first time in its *Diagnostic and Statistical Manual of Mental Disorders* (DSM). Binge-eating disorder was added to that list more recently.

Interestingly, the obesity epidemic began around the same time that eating disorder cases were peaking in the U.S. Over time, the societal pressure to be thin made way for the "big beautiful woman," or BBW, and the idea of *healthy obesity*, despite a consensus among the medical community that carrying extra weight is harmful.

Variations of addictive behavior occur along a spectrum. At one end are the compulsive exercisers and those obsessed with "clean" eating. At the opposite end, members of the fat acceptance movement are characterized by a different type of extreme. Rather than Instagramming pictures of their salad, these folks share memes celebrating laziness. Meanwhile, the middle ground remains sparse.

Whichever extreme you find yourself gravitating towards, you'll feel you're in good company. You'll find as much a cult-like devotion to doing too much as you will for doing too little. Among your kin, your addiction has been normalized...and therein lies the problem: comfort. This manifests itself in two ways. There's the physical comfort enjoyed by those in the sedentary extreme—the comfort of a couch, for example. That's the dopamine release, which requires longer and longer bouts of inactivity for the happiness derived from it to be sustained. This group is also at ease psychologically knowing that a lack of productivity is now acceptable in many circles.

Then there are the exercise addicts and those who adhere to militant diets. This group certainly isn't experiencing physical ease in their choice of endeavors but they too have found a tribe to validate their self-sabotaging ways. There's comfort in numbers, as the saying goes. This type of masochism is even celebrated among certain parts of society. How many times have we heard athletes being hailed as *heroes* for playing hurt?

Each extreme invites the possibility of illness and injury. Although still rare, the increased popularity of high-risk athletic pursuits has coincided with a rise in the number of cases of rhabdomyolysis. This life-threatening condition occurs when muscle fibers break down and leak toxic compounds into the blood, sometimes causing kidney damage. Indeed, it is possible to exercise yourself to death.

A more common result from overtraining and chronic dieting is adrenal burnout. Characterized by debilitating fatigue, impaired cognitive function, mood issues, and immune suppression, runners are particularly prone to the condition. If you're someone for whom laziness is the default, you may not have to worry about the dangers of over-exercising, but by shying away from exertion they also lose out on the benefits that come from periodic bouts of acute stress: a forced adaptation that results in greater resilience and an ability to better withstand and overcome adversity down the road. Of course, that's in addition to the serious health consequences associated with spending most of their lives sitting or lying down.

At the root of our drive for excess is our inherent inability to adopt a long-term view of our behaviors and their consequences. If our actions feel good in the here and now, that's enough for us. We're content. It can be uncomfortable to think beyond our current situation.

Plus, we're so often told to live in the present, and that may be wise in certain areas. However, just as your financial advisor would caution against a short-term investment strategy, psychology studies show that a long-term orientation leads to a more fulfilling and meaningful existence. But that involves too much effort. Extremes are far easier to comprehend. They're black and white. Moderation is the gray area. It's subject to interpretation, and we can't be bothered with its subtleties and distinctions.

DEFINING MODERATION

We hear it all the time, "everything in moderation." It's presented to us as if it's the master plan for a healthy, happy, successful existence. It sounds so simple, doesn't it? Clearly, though, there's a disconnect between understanding and implementing the moderate approach to health and fitness, as evidenced by increasing rates of obesity, chronic disease, and stress.

Here's the famous quote—most commonly attributed to Oscar Wilde—in its entirety:

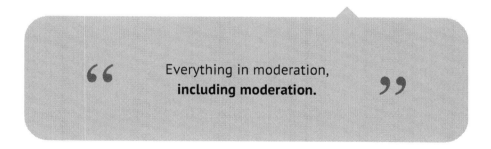

> " Everything in moderation,
> **including moderation.** "

That second part is almost always left out but that piece makes it much more instructive. The truth is, many of us use the moderation concept to rationalize unhealthy behaviors. Another issue with this approach is the subjective nature of it. How much is too much? Who gets to decide? In studies where participants are asked to gauge reasonable serving sizes of various food items, the responses are all over the place. Moderation for you might constitute excess for me or vice versa.

Can moderation ever be as sexy as extreme? I don't know, but if it's going to be, we need action steps to make the concept of moderation less vague and more relatable.

Here's what you can do on an individual level to help establish that middle ground in your wellness pursuits.

VARIETY

This is the key to slowing—or even preventing—hedonic adaptation. Keep things fresh to prevent boredom: Eat a varied diet; take a new exercise class. Cycling through a range of pleasurable activities will help you avoid habituation, or the diminished happiness response that occurs when the novelty of an experience dissipates.

DEFINE THE GOAL—IN TERMS OF HEALTH

Skinny isn't healthy. Skinny people get heart disease. Skinny people get cancer. Skinny people get diabetes.

AVOID HYPOCHONDRIA

We're living in the age of WebMD. We can Google our symptoms and we have a diagnosis at our fingertips within seconds. This is sometimes good but mostly bad, as it can trigger extreme behaviors. Instead, consult your own doctor to discuss your individual situation. Want to live longer? Use the Blue Zones as a guide. The term Blue Zones refers to geographic areas in which people have low rates of chronic disease and live longer than anywhere else. These populations move, but they don't participate in extreme sports; they eat well, but they don't starve themselves and then compensate with a binge. Bingeing devalues whatever the activity is anyway.

DROWN OUT THE ZEALOTS AND DISMISS THE DOGMA

This stuff feeds extreme behavior. Listen and learn but always consider context.

TAKE THE EMOTION OUT

Get some facts. More isn't even effective: A 2015 study in the *Journal of Health Psychology* showed that dieters take in more calories after a workout, so it's a wash.

STOP VIEWING FOOD AS BEING EITHER GOOD OR BAD

Instead, there are "always" foods and "sometimes" foods, just like we teach our children. This helps you avoid feelings of guilt and shame when you eat something forbidden.

DEATH TO DIETS

Fact: 95% of diets fail. Many who have suffered with eating disorders say the issue started as a diet, but got out of control. Banish the word.

ALLOW INDULGENCES

Adopt the 80/20 rule: Eat well 80% of the time and then indulge a bit with the other 20%. These should be planned, strategic cheats that give you something to look forward to. This has been shown to help with motivation and adherence. Pay attention to one thing: Do those occasional indulgences trigger a binge?

CHECK IN WITH YOURSELF

Question yourself, acknowledge how you're feeling. If you spend most of your time living in the extreme, what is it that draws you in that direction? Chip away until you discover those motivating factors.

LOOK FOR SIGNS OF OVERTRAINING

Tired? Sore? Dreading your next workout but still dragging yourself in? You should move every day but in the form of active recovery, a workout performed at a lower intensity and intended to increase blood flow, clear lactic acid, and manage soreness. Walking, stretching, yoga, and massage are examples.

LOOK FOR SIGNS OF FOOD OBSESSION

Constantly thinking about food? This is sometimes related to a nutrient deficiency, which can be tested for and then addressed with a more balanced eating plan and through the use of dietary supplements. Food obsession can lead to binge eating, so it may be necessary to physically remove yourself from certain situations where this is more likely to occur. Distract yourself with hobbies and other sources of happiness that don't involve food.

DON'T FIXATE ON ONE ASPECT

Even if your goal is purely aesthetic, your results don't hinge on one workout or one meal. It's the totality of all that you do that matters most. Whether it's a lean, muscular body you're after or a disease-free body, your goal requires a multi-pronged strategy. Obsessing over a single component means that an imbalance or deficiency will occur in some other area, and it will be that much harder to get where you want to be. How will going overboard in one area impact the equilibrium of the system as a whole?

MEDITATION AND OTHER FORMS OF MINDFULNESS

These were shown in a 2016 study at the University of California at San Francisco to help with recognizing hunger signals. At mealtime this means sitting down to eat, turning off electronic devices while eating, serving out individual portions, and chewing at least 20 times before swallowing. Rate your hunger on a scale of one to 10 to determine if you're eating out of boredom or stress. Don't wait until you're starving (1) to eat and stop once you're satisfied but not yet full (5 or 6).

DIGITAL DETOX

Social forums can be a source of inspiration, but avoid comparisons. When you start feeling envious of someone else's life, remind yourself that social media accounts are curated to show only the best. Don't be fooled. Even those who appear extremely happy in those photos have their share of challenges. By disconnecting for a set period of time, you'll add more hours back into your busy schedule and you'll stop holding yourself to someone else's standard for success.

YOU DON'T HAVE TO QUIT!

Realistically, if you're addicted to food or exercise, you're not going to suddenly begin abstaining. Instead, adapt and make some adjustments.

FEEDBACK DEVICES

These include heart rate variability (HRV) apps and devices, grip strength measurements, and sleep quality monitors. They can be valuable tools in terms of assessing recovery from a previous exercise session and preparedness for another one.

Moderation isn't always appropriate, and it too should be practiced within reason. Some of us can't stop at just one cookie, for example. If you have an addictive personality you may need to abstain completely.

It's easy to be moderate with things we don't like that much but we have a harder time mustering the willpower to resist stronger temptations. This is why it's so important to find something that works for you. My hope is that this book will serve as a template for doing just that.

Defining what a full life means requires some long-term thinking but it's also the key to finding that balance, that middle ground. A full life for most of us is one that includes lots of valuable experiences. The ones we crave because of the happiness they bring in both the short- and long-term and that are absent of physical pain, mental anguish, and internal negotiations. Loading up on these kinds of experiences will help crowd out the excesses and extremes.

In the words of Harvard psychologist Howard J. Shaffer, PhD:

> " As life becomes more worth living,
> the addiction loses influence. "

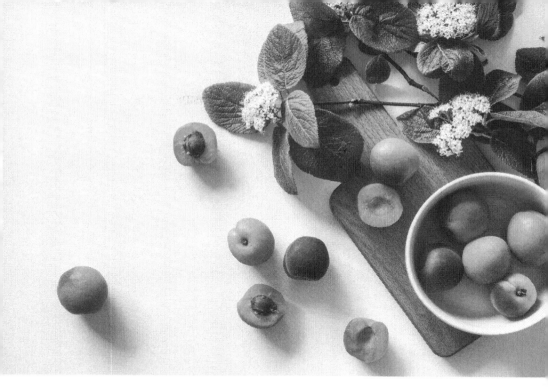

CHAPTER 02

Pillars of Vibrant Wellness: Diet, Exercise, Lifestyle

If you haven't already, you'll soon pick up on the overarching theme that ties together every chapter in this book. At the core of the *Urban Body Fix* program is the concept of personal responsibility. There are few areas in life over which we have as much control as we do over our health.

It is your duty—and yours alone—to support and protect your body and its amazingly complex and interdependent systems. Nobody's going to do it for you. Not me. Not your family. Not the government. Not even your doctor.

You can seek guidance and advice, but you own the choices you make regarding your health. This immense responsibility may seem intimidating to some, but it's also incredibly empowering. Blaming society, bad luck, or faulty DNA for your health woes is a futile and unproductive endeavor. Instead, let's channel that emotional energy into a more fulfilling and rewarding pursuit.

The title of this book could just as easily have been *Beyond Health*. While health is obviously something we strive for, many understand this term simply to mean the absence of disease, when true health actually encompasses so much more.

Unfortunately, the "healthy" label has also been hijacked by an industry that preys on unhappy people seeking quick fixes. Internet experts and others with questionable credentials peddle false hope and promote the idea that pleasure and contentment can be purchased.

I prefer the term "wellness" to embody not only the avoidance of illness but also a state of wholeness in which the individual thrives in every quality-of-life category. I refer to this type of wellness—and the kind of life it makes possible—as vibrant. It's a word we've all come across, but you really need to pause in order to appreciate its meaning. Here's a dictionary definition:

vi.brant /ˈvaɪbrənt/

(adj.)
1. full of energy and enthusiasm
2. pulsating with life, vigor, activity
3. energetic, exciting, and full of enthusiasm

OK, so it's actually a definition from each of three different dictionaries. I couldn't choose just one because all three are so powerful, and they perfectly capture what *Urban Body Fix* is all about. But how do we get there? And where do we start?

The current concept of self-care centers around technology. Many of those advances can be valuable tools. DNA testing, for example, can allow us to develop personalized diet and supplement protocols that make the most sense for us based on our own unique genetic makeup. This is exciting, and we should take full advantage of any opportunity to learn more about our bodies. Initially, though, this can be done in a much simpler way. By getting back to the basics, we avoid the mentality that wellness is too costly and too time-consuming, and therefore something that is out of our reach. Instead, let's focus on the fundamentals that will set us up for long-term, sustainable wellness in all areas. This requires a foundation, as well as an appreciation for how the different pieces of that foundation rely upon and integrate with one another.

In order for your body to work to its fullest potential, it is important to take into account all that it does for us. We need to return the favor and ensure we are providing our body with the best tools and supplies to work as a well-oiled machine. That involves positive change and powerful choices in health and in life. That's what we offer to our clients as well as to medical practices. Yes, we help individuals with overweight, fatigue, aching joints, and other ailments. But beyond pain relief, energy, and improved appearance—beyond the physical—we assist our clients to adjust their attitudes, transform their habits, and implement real, sustainable solutions that allow them to break free from American's current cycle of "sick care" and open a whole new world of wellness care. My hope is to do the same for you, the reader. That was my inspiration for writing this book, and it is what sustains me as I continue my work helping those interested in vibrant wellness.

This chapter is meant to give you the lay of the land as you prepare to start (or re-start) your quest toward more robust and vigorous living. If you've already begun that journey, perhaps you could benefit from some fine-tuning. It's based on my work with a wide range of clients over the past decade.

If you're wondering what's wrong with the current approach and why this paradigm shift is needed, here's your answer: America has a chronic disease problem. Consider these staggering statistics:

* 75% of Americans are overweight or obese, based on government health statistics.

* According to a report from the Centers for Disease Control and Prevention (CDC), 100 million Americans suffer from either diabetes or pre-diabetes. That equates to roughly half of all adults in the U.S.

* Data from the American Heart Association reveals that approximately 122 million of us have been diagnosed with heart disease, which kills 840,000 each year.

Together, these three health issues cost the economy nearly $2.5 trillion per year!

Now, the good news. Much of this suffering is preventable and, in some cases, even reversible. As it turns out, a poor diet is the number-one cause of death in the U.S. That was the finding of a 2018 article in the Journal of the American Medical Association. In fact, it's also the leading cause of mortality across the globe, attributable to more deaths than smoking. Why should these statistics give us hope? Because none of us have ever eaten anything by accident.

That brings us to our first, and most consequential, pillar of vibrant wellness. Most of the primary causes of chronic disease have been identified.

It's been estimated that about 90% **of heart disease cases,** 40% **of cancers, and** virtually all **diabetes diagnoses could be prevented with the right diet.**

But what exactly does that mean? Telling folks to "eat healthy" isn't very helpful, but such generic recommendations have been regurgitated for years via official government nutrition recommendations. The strategy hasn't been very effective, considering some of the statistics above.

A solid dietary foundation must be science-based. Research has pinpointed several mechanisms through which disease can develop in the body. There is a dietary component to each. Excess sugar, for example, can suppress the immune system, leaving us more vulnerable to infection by viruses and bacteria. Inflammation is a disease process that can cause plaque to deposit in the arteries, increasing the risk of a heart attack when the plaque ruptures and forms a blockage. We now know that overconsumption of the omega-6 fatty acids found in refined industrial seed oils (corn, soybean, cottonseed, peanut) can trigger this process. These oils—rampant in packaged foods—are still promoted as being healthy alternatives to more traditional cooking fats, despite mounting evidence to the contrary.

Many other foods are known to be protective. Compounds in berries and cruciferous vegetables, for example, can prevent the damage to a cell's DNA that could set the stage for a cancer diagnosis down the road. Fermented foods have long been known to strengthen the gut microbiome, home to 70% of our immune system. A more recent discovery was that those same friendly bacteria can even interact with the brain in a way that impacts mood. This is far from an exhaustive list. We will go into more detail on the role of diet and nutrition in a holistic wellness program later in the book.

How we eat is just as important as what we eat. The hustle and bustle of modern living often means eating on the run. Aside from increasing the risk of digestive issues, weight gain, heart disease, and diabetes, eating too quickly also takes away from what should be a pleasurable experience. In Spain and other European countries, meals sometimes last two hours, allowing time to savor every flavor and smell. Perhaps not coincidentally, these populations rate much higher than us on happiness scales.

Hydration is a component of overall nutrition that doesn't receive nearly enough attention. While we're taught in school that most of the human body is water, many of us still use thirst as an indicator of hydration status. Beyond maintaining fluid balance, water moves nutrients through the body and regulates our temperature. You may notice that your ability to focus suffers and you can't think as sharply when you're dehydrated. Your brain literally shrinks without adequate fluid intake.

It's clear that America in 2020 is an overfed and undernourished country. Eating is still seen by many as merely a way to procure energy rather than as the opportunity for nourishment and healing that it can be. The computer science acronym GIGO (garbage in, garbage out) is a fitting way to understand the effect this has on our health and performance. Ultra-processed foods make up the bulk of our grocery purchases. Common nutrient deficiencies lead to a sluggish metabolism, less energy and motivation for exercise, and other forms of physical activity, our second pillar of vibrant wellness.

Fitness is an $80 billion industry in the U.S. and growing steadily. Americans are clearly convinced of the importance of exercise but, unfortunately, that hasn't translated into improved health the way the experts tell us it's supposed to. What gives? We just touched on one of the problems: We don't fuel ourselves properly. We're overweight because we don't exercise enough, but we don't exercise enough because we're overweight.

If we could look inside our bodies and witness the short- and long-term exercise-induced repair processes that take place on a cellular and metabolic level, we probably wouldn't shy away from physical endeavors as much as we do. But when our primary motivation to run, lift, sweat, and burn comes in the form of extrinsic factors, we quickly become dissatisfied.

Surveys show that the vast majority of Americans who begin an exercise program quit within a few months of starting. Unfortunately, sporadic, infrequent bouts of exercise don't provide nearly as powerful a benefit as the consistent variety required for vibrant wellness.

A mindset shift is needed from aesthetic goals to those related to performance. I define fitness as the process of making everything we do outside of exercise and elsewhere in life, easier, safer, and more comfortable. As you may relate, being tight, stiff, and sore can have a pretty detrimental effect on one's quality of life.

Aside from the physical benefits, exercise also teaches discipline. Once you've reexamined your exercise goals, you'll establish habits and routines that get reinforced as you continue to see and feel progress. You'll discover what works and what doesn't. These rules will provide structure and stability to your life, which will transfer to the other pillars—diet and lifestyle.

So what do we mean by lifestyle? The short answer is anything that isn't diet and exercise, but with the primary focus on emotional and psychological wellness. Leading a relaxed, stress-free life is a lot harder than it sounds. We all have busy schedules, and we tend to spread ourselves too thin. This "run yourself ragged" existence isn't sustainable in the long-run. It can have negative effects on your overall health, especially your immunity.

Researchers have found that when a person is more stressed out, their immune response is suppressed. Stress and anxiety don't just affect the mind, but the body as well. If your body is being over-exhausted and stressed by exertion, your immune response to unwanted germs and pathogens can be less effective. This is a reminder of how neglecting one of the three pillars can lead to an imbalance in another that throws the entire system out of whack.

You could be eating the cleanest diet and have the most effective exercise program, but if you're harboring unhealthy emotions, you'll find it much harder to achieve vibrant wellness. Anger, resentment, and other negative feelings serve as a distraction. They sap your energy, creativity, and focus.

Positivity, on the other hand, leads to poise, determination, and courage. This type of well-being manifests itself in our minds and carries over to our wellness pursuits in the physical realm. Positive thoughts make it easier to build and sustain healthy eating habits and fitness routines, for example. This is just another example of how the three pillars are interdependent, with each relying on the others to support and stabilize the foundation.

Emotional wellness involves acknowledging, understanding, and communicating your feelings in constructive ways. In the process, you'll develop and sharpen the coping skills you need to adapt to and overcome life's stressors. Beyond creating inner calm, this resilience allows you to navigate the obstacles that may prevent you from sticking to the healthy diet and exercise habits you've implemented or intend to implement. In fact, being in touch with your emotions can help you to predict and preempt any potential hurdle before the possibility of retreat can even enter the equation.

Social well-being is a crucial but overlooked aspect of healthy living. Inhabitants of the Blue Zones—parts of the world with the highest concentration of centenarians—enjoy a strong sense of community, one of several shared traits thought to explain the impressive longevity of these groups. Healthy relationships promote feelings of self-worth and provide a support system during trying times. Further highlighting the interconnectedness of the three pillars are studies showing that social well-being lowers the risk of Alzheimer's disease and stroke.

Another component of the lifestyle pillar is that of spirituality, a set of deeply personal values and beliefs that gives us a sense of purpose in life. Unlike religion, spirituality is more of an individual practice, though the two are related in that each offers us meaning beyond the material world. Both religion and spirituality—defined in various ways depending on the person—have been associated with increased happiness in research studies.

Another clue emerges from the Blue Zone populations in the longevity puzzle: intellectual wellness. While it's often assumed that memory loss and impaired cognitive function are inevitable consequences of getting older, observations of the longest-living people on the planet prove that brain aging is multifactorial. Mentally stimulating activities such as word games, chess, and puzzles are known to activate specialized neurons and increase production of *new* brain cells—even in older adults. Crafts, music, and other hobbies that involve creativity have been shown to exert similar effects.

Sleep and relaxation fall into the lifestyle category as well. (We will go more in depth on each later in the book.) Relaxation techniques help with sleep and stress issues, both of which impact your success with diet and exercise protocols. Detect a theme yet?

Poor sleep hygiene—assessed in terms of both duration and quality—can obviously mean less energy for exercise. What is not so obvious is how a sleep deficit can make it harder to stick to a healthy eating plan. As it turns out, sleep is when our bodies produce hormones, some of which are involved in hunger signaling. Fewer hours of sleep are associated with increased cravings and weight gain. High-tech gadgets and gizmos from the nascent "sleep technology" market promise the best slumber of our lives. But amber-hued glasses, smart pillows, and cooling pads don't address the underlying cause of insomnia but are merely reflective of our culture's increased expectations of a Band-Aid fix.

The relaxation industry does a better job at root-cause healing, and more Americans are convinced of the need for de-stressing. More of us, unfortunately, are also still seeking out the pharmaceutical approach. Relaxation techniques don't just relax, though. They declutter and strengthen the mind, teaching self-discipline and adaptability. Exercise and other forms of physical activity play a complementary role here.

The problem with most diet and weight loss books (which this is *not*!) is their focus on an external image or outward perception of health. They promise a certain look—often based on societal standards—but this isn't wellness. Even "healthy living" resources often leave us with the impression that we can weigh, measure, or count our way to happiness, and that looking good equates with feeling good.

Remember the personal responsibility piece? That means making holistic wellness a priority and staying informed. Our website and social media channels can help with that. With your pillars in place, you're equipped to evaluate and implement information in this rapidly evolving industry as you see fit.

When embarking on the journey toward wellness, it's easy to feel overwhelmed. Self-help gurus throw so much information at us, we assume we've got to implement every single change right away, we soon become discouraged, and we throw our hands up. That's because there's little or no focus on building a foundation.

That foundation is what keeps you centered. It's what you return to after you've strayed—and you will, and that's OK. You'll be tested, you'll be tempted, and life will get in the way at times. As long as those pillars have been established, though, you'll find their pull to be so magnetic that outside influence stands little chance.

Another difference between UBF and other healthy living "how-to" manuals you may have come across: There's no dogma or zealotry here. Notice I didn't prescribe a specific diet or exercise program. Sure, I'll make recommendations. With diet, for example, most Americans would benefit from a focus on healthy fats and low glycemic carbohydrate sources to fuel the body. When possible, I advise limiting the intake of conventional meat, dairy, and produce and opting for organic. Doing so will prevent the accumulation of toxic chemicals in our tissues. When it comes to exercise, I stress consistency and the need for you to challenge yourself. Other than that, I just want you to move!

Getting too caught up in the minutiae is counterproductive. Balance is critical to making these lifestyle modifications sustainable over the long term. So within the basic parameters laid out in this chapter and throughout this book, you've got freedom and flexibility to make wellness your own.

I want you to do it your way.
You have to do it your way.

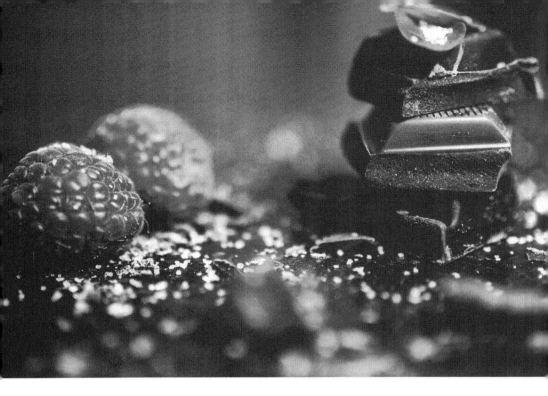

CHAPTER 03

Feed Me!

How to Interpret What Your Cravings Are Telling You

So you're on board with the *Urban Body Fix* philosophy, you understand the importance of moderation, and your pillars are in place. What's next? Now, you're ready for the nuts-and-bolts of the program. But first, you'll need to know how to respond to one of the most common pitfalls on the path to vibrant wellness.

While proponents of extreme dieting suggest we silence our food cravings, this approach doesn't play out very well in the real world. A strategy of deny-and-deprive may work for a week or two, but this quest for perfection almost always leads to abandonment of the diet.

Cravings are not something to be ignored, as they give us a valuable read on our nutritional status and psychological state. This feedback can help us understand and anticipate the body's needs and wants, and prevent them from derailing our journey toward holistic wellness.

WHAT ARE CRAVINGS?

It's important to distinguish between cravings and hunger. For years, we've been advised to "eat less and exercise more" if we want to lose weight. In the short-term, this approach creates a caloric deficit and may indeed help you drop a few pounds. Soon, though, your body adapts to this new metabolic set point. Results then stall unless you drop your calories even lower.

Traditional dieting is characterized by a generalized, near-constant, and sometimes ravenous hunger. This is a physiological state with a clearly identifiable cause: reduced caloric intake, increased activity level, or a combination of the two. True hunger is often accompanied by other symptoms beyond a grumbling tummy:

* Headache

* Dizziness

* Nausea

* Mood issues

* Brain fog

It's important to note that thirst is sometimes mistaken for hunger. Obviously, eating when you're actually dehydrated can lead to weight gain. While hunger and thirst cues can overlap, the latter is commonly associated with these additional symptoms:

* Dry skin and eyes

* Low energy

* Muscle cramps

* Dark urine

Understanding why and how we get hungry is fairly straightforward, but the development and manifestation of cravings can be multifactorial and, therefore, more complicated. And though hunger is almost exclusively viewed through the prism of weight management, cravings can be indicative of underlying health issues. Getting to the bottom of them may require some detective work.

TYPES OF CRAVINGS

These intense hankerings for specific foods are incredibly common, affecting 97% of women and 68% of men, according to one study. Our cravings tend to fall into several categories, which often overlap with one another.

HORMONAL

When you think of food cravings, do you picture an expectant mom devouring a pint of cookie-dough ice cream or a box of red velvet cupcakes? Cravings during pregnancy are usually caused by a drop in dopamine, a brain chemical responsible for feelings of pleasure.

Estrogen and progesterone are the primary hormones involved in common premenstrual syndrome (PMS) symptoms, which include intense urges for specific foods, usually of the salty and sugary variety. These cravings tend to occur later in the menstrual cycle, as progesterone counters the appetite-suppressant effects of estrogen.

Low serotonin levels can increase cravings for sweets in both genders. Low levels of this neurotransmitter are associated with depression and anxiety. Sugar and other high-glycemic carbohydrates provide a quick mood boost, a feeling that the brain commits to memory, which explains our inclination for these types of treats during times of stress.

Leptin is a hormone made in the fat cells, which then travels to the brain to tell it we've had enough to eat and that our energy stores have been filled. When this system is functioning properly, the brain will then flip the switch on hunger and shut down our desire to eat. Sometimes, things get out of whack, and the brain no longer receives that signal. That's when appetite and cravings persist. Even though we've just eaten, our brain thinks we're starving! This condition is called leptin resistance.

The other *hunger hormone*, ghrelin, also influences our food cravings. Produced in the gut, ghrelin signals to the brain that we're hungry. Extreme dieters and others on restricted eating plans have higher levels of circulating ghrelin, which stimulates appetite and increases food intake, especially in the form of complex carbohydrates and starches. In turn, these individuals find it harder to lose weight. Interestingly, ghrelin levels appear to increase more at night, which is also when intense cravings are more likely to occur.

Although not technically considered hormones, endorphins also act on the part of the brain responsible for pleasure and reward. These chemicals are the body's natural painkillers and have been linked to addictive behavior. Acting in a similar way to morphine, endorphins trigger a "runner's high" or a state of euphoria after sex. When endorphin levels drop, we tend to crave fatty foods.

Sugar has an opiate-like effect that we just can't expect from vegetables. The impact is so powerful that it leads to increased cravings and, often, food addiction. Similar to illicit drugs, tolerance can develop, necessitating increasing amounts of these pleasure-inducing substances in order to achieve a feeling similar to that initial "high."

EMOTIONAL

Unlike hunger, cravings have more to do with our emotional needs rather than with a demand for physical sustenance. A craving for spicy food, for example, may reflect a desire for adventure and excitement, while a hankering for ice cream may be tied to the joy of a childhood memory and nostalgia for a simpler time. Crunchy snacks may offer an outlet when we're enraged, starchy foods can provide comfort during periods of uncertainty and chocolate connotes love and affection when we are lonely. Indulging in these and other "naughty" foods are an opportunity to assert our independence and to challenge authority.

This form of self-medication takes place without us knowing. Its cycle can quickly spin out of control. Our cravings often mask subconscious negativity, which will fester if left untended. Untangling and translating these urges can give us insight into our emotional health, a key component of vibrant wellness.

NUTRITIONAL

Do our food cravings correspond to nutrients that the body may be lacking? This was the prevailing theory for many years and likely originated with research on pica, an eating disorder that causes cravings for non-food substances, such as dirt, ice, clay, and paint chips. Pica is more common among children and pregnant women, two groups at greater risk for deficiencies in minerals such as iron and zinc.

In the 18th century, it was observed that British sailors were experiencing intense cravings for fruit. It was later determined that these men had been suffering from scurvy, a severe vitamin C deficiency.

A craving for chocolate is often pegged to a need for magnesium, an essential mineral found in cacao. Cravings for meat are sometimes attributed to a lack of iron or protein in the diet. A desire for savory foods could be indicative of a sodium deficiency which, although not common among the general population, is a concern for older adults, athletes, and those taking certain medications.

While most cravings are psychological or environmental in nature, it is plausible that some stem from a nutrient deficiency. This theory continues to be debated, but it does seem to apply to specific populations or certain periods when a lack of key vitamins and minerals is known to be more common.

CAUSES OF CRAVINGS

Satisfying your hunger can be as simple as filling your belly with whatever is accessible. Cravings, however, are much more specific in nature. The types of cravings we experience are largely dictated by the cause, of which there are many.

STRESS

There's a reason we reach for unhealthy foods during times of stress and anxiety. Researchers have determined that sugar in particular can alter production of the stress hormone cortisol, as well as the function of the hippocampus. These changes somehow impact the way the brain interprets and responds to various stressors. Sugar also boosts serotonin levels, which can induce feelings of pleasure and relaxation.

POOR SLEEP

Many of our hormones are released during sleep. A sleep deficit is associated with an increase in ghrelin and a drop in leptin, a situation that leads to constant hunger. According to the research in this area, even one night of poor sleep can have this effect.

Through a different mechanism, sleep deprivation increases levels of endocannabinoid. This is the same system that triggers what some marijuana users refer to as the "munchies." In this state, we specifically crave hyperpalatable foods like cookies and chips.

Additional research has shown that a lack of sleep sharpens the olfactory system, enhancing the effect that food aromas have on the brain. The result is a series of mixed signals that make the brain vulnerable to alluring smells—more along the lines of a freshly baked muffin rather than a bowl of steamed broccoli!

EXTERNAL FACTORS

There's no question that cultural, ethnic, and religious factors impact how we look at food. These and other aspects of our lives, such as our jobs, can be all-encompassing. Some would argue that they exert a more powerful effect on our cravings than any physiological or psychological component.

Society's obsession with body weight and other established cultural norms certainly play a role in shaping how we look at cravings. In certain situations, indulgences are thought to be justified. Foods typically associated with feelings of guilt or shame are suddenly deemed OK, and this sometimes leads to binging.

During pregnancy, for example, there's a built-in societal approval to eat foods we otherwise might not. The justification is that we're "eating for two," when in reality a pregnant woman only requires an extra 300 calories per day when carrying a child. In contrast, women in many other parts of the world maintain their traditional diet during pregnancy.

According to one study, women born in other countries don't experience cravings for chocolate during their menstrual cycle the way those born in the U.S. do. Researchers have concluded that this is a "culture-bound construct" unique to North America and that those not born here are less likely to think of the menstrual cycle as the cause of—or excuse for—indulging.

GIVE IN—SOMETIMES!

It's important to make clear that cravings are natural. And normal! Just make sure that whatever you choose to indulge in actually does scratch the itch. If you're craving ice cream, for example, a *light* version probably isn't going to do it for you. Your body is smarter than that. Have the real thing and then move on. When indulging, however, keep in mind the lessons of Chapter 1 on moderation. When indulgences become a daily affair, they are no longer indulgences.

If your cravings have gotten out of control—and you've addressed some of the causative factors above—there are several strategies you can use to defuse the situation.

- Try real-food substitutions (synthetic or impostor treats will be recognized as such by both brain and body). A craving for potato chips may be satisfied by a handful of salted almonds or cashews. If you're jonesing for some candy, first try some dried fruit and the natural sugar it contains. Longing for a soda? Try a naturally-flavored carbonated beverage or a brand of soda sweetened with a natural sugar alternative like stevia (I like the Zevia brand). If your hankering for chocolate is indicative of a magnesium deficiency, try taking a daily magnesium supplement, which provides a host of other health benefits. But perhaps a couple of squares of truly dark chocolate (80% cacao or above) will do the trick. The brands I enjoy are Theo, Equal Exchange, Pascha, or Green & Black's. A naturally sweetened sugar-free variety is Lily's.

- Depending on your personality, the cause of your cravings, and your health status and fitness goals, it may be necessary to restrict sugar completely. This strategy has been shown to eliminate cravings for sweets over time, as our tastebuds adjust.

- Journaling our triggers can help to identify potentially problematic situations and to be more proactive in avoiding them in the future. Be specific in noting exactly which emotions you're experiencing when cravings hit and what is going on in your life at that moment.

- Limiting refined carbohydrates and excess fructose in the diet may also help, as both are known to lead to leptin resistance by raising triglycerides in a process similar to insulin resistance.

- While natural sugar alternatives like stevia, erythritol, and monk fruit can make for healthy swaps, avoid artificial sweeteners. These chemicals—sucralose, aspartame, and acesulfame potassium—can disrupt gut bacteria and alter brain chemistry in a way that actually *increases* cravings.

- Getting creative in the kitchen can make a bland, boring diet more exciting, helping to decrease the likelihood of straying. You've got a spice rack, time to use it!

- Among its many other benefits, regular exercise prevents leptin resistance.

- Dietary fat suppresses ghrelin, as does a higher protein intake, especially when starting with breakfast.

- Sometimes you need a change of scenery. When temptation strikes, distract yourself with a bath or shower, or a walk outdoors. Call a friend. Just leave the situation.

- Exercise, sex, and massage can all increase endorphins without the need for food.

- Whenever possible, stick to whole, unprocessed foods. While shakes, bars, and packaged meal replacements certainly have their place, they are refined and more quickly digested. As such, it doesn't register with the brain that you've just eaten.

- Chewing gum or sucking on a mint has been shown to suppress cravings, perhaps due to the relaxation-inducing effects of peppermint. Brushing your teeth right after eating can trick the brain into thinking you're beginning your bedtime routine and that the "kitchen" is now closed.

- A consistent meal schedule can help crowd out opportunities for indulgences.

- Mindfulness. We will get into much greater detail on relaxation techniques later in the book but, for now, understand that breathing exercises—before *and* during meals—and the awareness they help to create can prevent mindless eating.

There's a reason most diets fail. You'd probably agree that eating is one of the greatest pleasures in life. Living with a list of forbidden foods in your head is a miserable existence. Science has made it very clear that a balanced diet is the most sensible approach for both weight management and disease prevention. On a day-to-day basis, it can also eliminate the distraction posed by food cravings.

Learning to interpret your cravings goes along with what we've covered thus far in the book. As the owner of your body, it is your responsibility to stay attuned to its needs and wants via cravings and other indicators. While you continue reading, it will be helpful to think about how some of the mind-body strategies we discuss can be used to address your food cravings, as well as any other addictive behaviors you may be practicing that may be barriers in your quest for vibrant wellness.

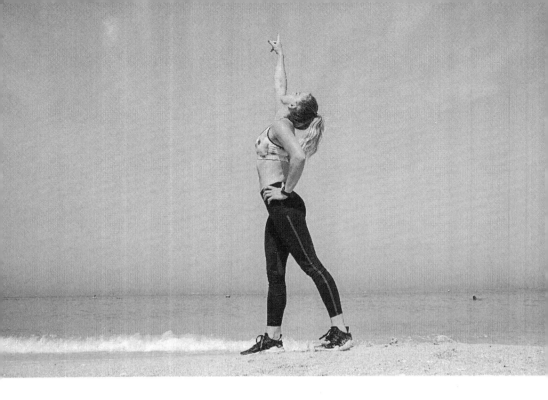

CHAPTER 04

Move That Body,
What's Your Jam for Exercise?

If you're hoping I'm about to reveal the best Tabata program for torching fat or the fastest way to a bubble butt, you may be disappointed. The truth is, I'm still in search of both.

Instead, this section of the book will be devoted to helping you redefine exercise, refocus your fitness efforts, and most importantly, chip away at the most common barriers preventing you from getting regular physical activity.

The buy-in doesn't seem to be the issue. In fact, Americans appear to be more convinced than ever of the benefits of exercise. In one survey, 69% of respondents said they believed that regular exercise would help them to drop bad habits.

Yet, additional research has revealed that only 23% of us meet the recommended guidelines for physical activity, and nearly half of those who begin an exercise routine quit within six months.

So what gives? Why does the U.S. continue to rank as one of the laziest countries, despite spending over $10 billion per year on exercise equipment? What is getting in the way of us maintaining a level of fitness sufficient to reap its proven benefits?

We know from surveys what some of the obstacles are. And, if we care enough, we also know how to get around them.

THE BARRIER: *I DON'T HAVE TIME*

Too little time is commonly cited as the biggest reason so many of us don't exercise more. It's true, Americans in 2020 are an overworked bunch. Our fast-paced, frenetic lifestyles have come to define our modern culture. On average, we have a mere 89 minutes of free time per day, according to surveys.

Strangely, many of us view *busyness* as a source of pride, a badge of honor. We associate long hours with higher status. As long as our always-on-the-go speed of life and our drive to have it all is celebrated, work-life balance may be non-existent.

Unless...

Research shows that the average American spends two hours and 24 minutes each day on social media and 2.8 hours watching television. Still think you don't have time to work out?

Exercise doesn't have to eat into all of our leisure time. Although, some of us have become convinced that exercise doesn't *work* unless you can devote countless hours to it each week, research tells a different story.

A 2016 study, for example, showed that a 10-minute sprint interval session was as effective as a 50 minute workout at improving several measures of cardiovascular and metabolic function. Mounds of additional research have further confirmed that short, intense bouts of physical activity are as effective—and, in some cases superior—to longer duration exercise such as running. A 2009 study even found that interval training increases testosterone and human growth hormone.

The weight management benefits of interval training can be attributed to excess post-exercise oxygen consumption, or EPOC. This refers to the work your body has to do after a workout to restore homeostasis. The *afterburn* effect is far more significant in response to high-intensity interval training (H.I.I.T.) than for steady-state exercise, where the majority of the caloric expenditure occurs *during* the activity.

Thanks to EPOC, your metabolism is elevated for 24-48 hours after your workout has ended, even if the rest of your day is spent on the couch binge-watching your favorite Netflix series. As it turns out, most of the calories we burn throughout the day have nothing to do with our gym time, and instead are part of our resting metabolic rate (RMR). Accounting for up to 75% of daily caloric expenditure, RMR includes the normal bodily processes required to keep us alive, like respiration and digestion, as well as recovery from exercise.

Activities like sprinting and resistance training have a more profound and lasting impact on RMR than those that involve less intensity. These forms of exercise are incredibly time-efficient, but what if HIIT isn't an option for you, either because of an injury or a medical condition? How can you boost your RMR on a tight schedule?

In 2012, researchers at the Healthy Lifestyles Research Center at Arizona State University reported that three 10-minute workout sessions were more effective than a single, continuous 30-minute session in terms of lowering blood pressure. The exercise of choice in this study was a brisk walk, performed at 75% of the participants' maximum heart rate.

A previous study, this one on children, found that bouts of exercise as short as five minutes in duration improved the cholesterol profiles of the participants as well as an extended session. Earlier research demonstrated an advantage of intermittent exercise for weight loss compared to a longer workout. Such a fitness program would produce more frequent *jolts* to the metabolism, resulting in a more dramatic, cumulative effect.

The researchers call this fractitionized exercise but we'll call them fitness *snacks*. More sustainable over the long-term than a commitment to exercise classes or gym sessions, this approach to fitness can be incorporated throughout the average workday. You've heard this advice before: take the stairs rather than the elevator, park your car further from the building, go for a walk on your lunch break. Such activity falls into the category of non-exercise activity thermogenesis, or NEAT. These are the calories you burn doing anything other than eating, sleeping, or exercising— everything from fidgeting and house work to pacing and chewing gum. Yes, these activities count. No, they won't make you an athlete, but most of us aren't training for the Iron Man.

In the world of college and professional sports, an athlete's year is broken down into phases, each characterized by varying degrees of exercise frequency and intensity. This is called periodization. High-volume training blocks never last more than a couple of months and are followed by a period of "deloading," during which training sessions are scaled back. Athletic trainers design programs in such a way so that the athlete is in peak condition at just the right time. The lesson for the rest of us? More is not better, not even for a gifted competitor. Later in the book we will discuss the role of cortisol, a stress hormone that is beneficial in small doses but counterproductive when produced in excess. Overtraining can result in the adrenal glands pumping out too much cortisol, leading to a suppressed immune system. Cortisol can also increase cravings, specifically for snack foods and those high in sugar and fat. In a sense, then, too much exercise can make us fat!

Many Americans report that a lack of motivation keeps them from exercising more regularly. Part of the problem is how fitness has been sold to us over the years. If you've been convinced that exercise has to be a grueling, back-breaking endeavor, then it's understandable that it might not be near the top of your to-do list.

It doesn't help when we're bombarded with images of stick-thin cover models and superhero physiques. This makes fitness seem like something reserved for the wealthy or the genetically gifted. *No pain, no gain* is still the standard for some, making us mere mortals feel that society's ideal is unattainable. Obsessing over strictly aesthetic pursuits makes the entire process seem overwhelming. Many of us then decide the effort is pointless.

If motivation is an issue for you then perhaps your goals are too broad or too generic. This is often why so many New Year's resolutions fail. Research shows that having a very specific goal makes it easier to stay on track. Aiming to lose 20 pounds is setting yourself up for failure. You need to lose five pounds before you can lose 20, right? Breaking up ambitious goals into smaller, more achievable steps will make the process seem less daunting. Celebrate the small victories along the way and you'll generate the momentum and confidence to continue moving forward.

Using the wrong metrics is another form of self-sabotage. Scale weight provides an instructive example. Many of us are obsessed with this number. But the scale isn't a very accurate indicator of health and fitness, nor does it tell us very much about our progress. The scale weighs everything: fat, muscle, bone, internal organs, gut bacteria, and even your feces. Your scale weight fluctuates—not only from one day to the next, but also throughout the same day—based on water consumption, carbohydrate and sodium intake, activity level, and hormone function. Weight loss almost always involves some muscle breakdown, which slows your metabolism and leads to weight *gain* over the long-term. Fat loss is what you really want.

If you've fallen into a similar trap, you might be more successful focusing on a specific health outcome. There's nothing wrong with wanting to sculpt a curvier booty or hoping to "see your abs" by summer. What good is any of that, though, if you drop dead of a heart attack at age 47?

The potential physique-enhancing effects of exercise are pretty well-accepted. However, bulging biceps and six-pack abs aren't a priority for many of us. Nearly all Americans, though, would like to move better throughout the day, avoid injury, and live as long as possible free of disease.

It may help to change your mindset and try getting excited about the health-promoting effects that regular exercise can offer. Americans are suffering. Most of us have at least one chronic disease and pain is one of the biggest reasons for doctors visits. Exercise can help with these and many other issues. One study found that a daily 25 minute brisk walk can repair DNA damage, and add seven years to our lives!

If your motivation is waning because you think your physique goals are out of reach, try immersing yourself in the proven wellness benefits of exercise. Here are just some of the many health conditions that can be managed with regular exercise:

* High blood pressure

* Certain cancers

* Diabetes

* Anxiety

* Depression

* Chronic fatigue syndrome

* Osteoporosis

* Fibromyalgia

* Erectile dysfunction

The cool part is this: by focusing on health-oriented goals, you'll still improve your physique in the process. Some of the same exercises that lower heart disease risk, for example, will also help you to tighten and tone some of your problem areas.

Sports psychologists have studied the underlying intrinsic factors that drive athletic endeavors. Their research has shown that friendly competition is a stronger motivator than support from friends and family, at least in the context of our interactions online. Beach Body Challenge, Healthy Wage, and Diet Bet are just a few of the many online body transformation contests and fitness challenges that may appeal to an individual with a competitive streak. Many of these offer financial incentives as well, and this tactic is also known to improve adherence.

The experts have other tips for getting—and staying—motivated to exercise. For starters, you can try working out first thing in the morning. If you put it off until later in the day, something else might come up. Also, our willpower tends to dip with each passing hour and you may be more tempted to blow off your exercise session as the day progresses.

Look at your workout as an appointment—with yourself, a partner, a trainer, or instructor. Block it off in your calendar as you would a trip to the dentist or a dinner date.

To recap: only once you've defined your goal can you summon the necessary drive. Maybe you want to get off your meds, have more energy, or sleep better. Whatever it may be, find your spark and keep your eyes on the prize.

And those days on which your lack of motivation is especially debilitating? Just tell yourself that all you have to do is get to the door—of the gym, the yoga studio, the racquet club. Once you're there it's highly unlikely that you'll turn around and head back home. You'll go inside and *something* will happen. Remember, you don't have to get into beast mode every time you work out. Exercise in all forms is an antidepressant. You might not hit a PR, but you'll leave with a rush of mood-boosting endorphins to get you through the rest of your day.

One caveat: Having a love-hate relationship with exercise is normal, but if you're dragging yourself into the gym or if you've been dreading your workout all week long, drop it and find something you enjoy a bit more. That leads us to our next point.

Some folks just don't like exercise. Or, at least, what they assume exercise to be.

Stereotypes abound: *Lifting weights is for meatheads. Running will destroy my knees. Yoga is for hippies. Squats are dangerous.* The list goes on and the discouragement and close-mindedness continues.

As we touched on above, many of us—to our detriment—still view exercise through the prism of changing our appearance. This mentality stems from pervasive societal stigmas and rampant body-shaming. Self-consciousness, fear of embarrassment, and past negative experiences can also shape our views of what it means to exercise.

THE URBAN BODY FIX: RE-DEFINE IT

Exercise is whatever you want it to be and you've got more options than ever before, from baby goat yoga to skijoring and everything in between. You can choose a different modality every day for a year and never repeat the same workout twice. Enjoy being outside? Rent a kayak or go horseback riding. If the social element increases adherence for you, then join a class.

If you need a push or a personalized routine, hire a personal trainer, a service that is now offered online for use with your living room, basement, or garage set-up. While we're on the subject of home-based workouts, there are hundreds of apps and streaming options that may appeal to the introverts out there.

Variety isn't just the spice of life, it's actually crucial to preventing burnout and avoiding overuse injuries. Keeping things fresh also ensures you continue to see results. Your body is smart. It figures out and adapts to whatever you throw at it. If you keep performing the same exercise, the same way, it's only a matter of time before you reach a plateau.

Variety can be as simple as switching your yoga routine from vinyasa to ashtanga. At the gym, you can spend a few weeks using lighter weights for higher repetitions to focus more on muscular endurance. Or try using a wider stance the next time you squat. You'll emphasize different parts of the same muscles and probably trigger some new muscle growth in those previously-neglected areas. To hit your core in a different way, replace your usual sit-up routine with some Pilates. Simply changing the route of your morning jog can also prevent boredom.

These are just a few examples. As they say, the best workout is the one you're not currently doing! If you're an exercise novice, you can actually expect to see more results and faster compared to someone for whom the training stimulus is no longer new and whose body has long-ago adapted.

For many of us, simply spending more time in a standing position can go a long way toward improving our health. Depending on the study, Americans sit for anywhere from 10 to 13 hours each day. In a recent study, 9.5 hours of sitting was associated with a "statistically significant increased risk of death." While I won't try to convince you that "sitting is the new smoking," there is a growing list of potential ailments linked to our increasingly sedentary lifestyles:

- Decreased blood flow to the brain and a corresponding risk of cognitive impairment, anxiety, and depression

- Postural issues

- Tight hip flexor muscles and a reduced range of motion

- Inactive abdominal muscles and a resulting accumulation of fat around the waist

- An increased risk of osteoporosis from weakening bones

There's no one-size-fits-all approach to exercise. Anything that gets you moving will be beneficial, both in the short- and long-term.

THE BARRIER: *I'M TOO OLD*

In one survey, more than 2 in 5 respondents said they were too old for exercise. The average age at which they began to feel that way? Forty-one!

Hormone changes and a more sluggish metabolism are realities that a middle-aged exerciser will have to work around but those certainly aren't deal-breakers. And yes, it's even more important for older adults to warm up properly and to avoid high impact movements but the investment is worth it when you consider the results of a 2018 study in the journal *Neurology*. The researchers found that "very fit" middle-aged women were 88% less likely to develop dementia. Older adults who engage in resistance training also suffer fewer falls. Even in those who have never previously exercised the development of disease if prolonged once they begin a regular workout routine. In the words of the researchers, those who are fittest in middle age experience "compressed morbidity," meaning they spend less time ill or disabled. In other words, they're not just living longer, they're living better.

THE URBAN BODY FIX: REALITY CHECK

Julia Hawkins might not be a household name but in 2017, at the age of 101, she became the oldest competitor in the history of the USA Track and Field Outdoor Masters Championship. Two years later, at 103, Julia won the gold medal in the 100-meter dash at the National Senior Games, with a time of 46.07 seconds. In her words:

> As you get older, you need challenges...they keep you alive.

Now obviously, older adults and those with certain health issues should receive medical clearance from their doctor before starting an exercise program. Exercise prescriptions should take into account one's injury history and appropriate modifications should be made. The good news is that even light exercise can be beneficial. In fact, a 2019 article in the *British Medical Journal* listed washing dishes as one of many activities associated with longevity.

The gentle, flowing movements that characterize tai chi and qi gong are particularly well-suited to elderly individuals. Studies conducted at Harvard University have demonstrated that these activities can strengthen muscles, improve balance and coordination, and reduce stress. They've even been found to complement more traditional therapies used in fighting conditions such as chronic fatigue syndrome, depression, and Parkinson's disease. The proof is certainly in the pudding when it comes to these ancient martial arts techniques. They've been practiced for thousands of years in China, which tends to have lower disease rates than the U.S. and in Hong Kong, which currently has the longest life expectancy of any country in the world.

PROGRESSION, NOT PERFECTION—KEEP MOVING FORWARD

If exercise were a pill, we'd all be taking it. But exercise is actually better than a pill: low-risk, high-reward. Countless studies have demonstrated the life-extending and life-enhancing benefits of regular physical activity. Don't think of it as exercise if you'd prefer not to. Simply aim for a more active life, doing things that you enjoy and getting better at them.

The goal: move more, sit less.

Shift your thinking from how you look to how you perform and your fitness journey will be a rewarding and fulfilling one.

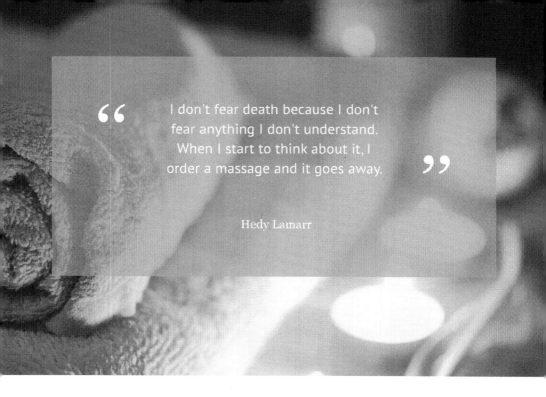

> I don't fear death because I don't fear anything I don't understand. When I start to think about it, I order a massage and it goes away.

Hedy Lamarr

CHAPTER 05

Work that Body! Massage

Okay, so I may be biased but I felt this topic deserved its own chapter. As a licensed massage therapist, I've witnessed firsthand the powerful therapeutic effects of this ancient practice. Once seen as a guilty pleasure, massage is now firmly entrenched as one of the most effective drug-free methods of physical rehabilitation and psychological rejuvenation in alternative medicine. It's also a popular complementary therapy, increasingly used alongside more conventional treatments for a host of medical issues.

Massage therapy is no longer an indulgence; it's yet another opportunity to invest in your short- and long-term wellness. Along with the many other modalities discussed throughout this book, massage has earned its place in the *Urban Body Fix* toolkit for those of us focused on the emerging concept of healthspan. Obviously, we want to live as long as possible but, more importantly, we hope to live well in those extra years, remaining productive, pain-free, and vibrant.

Over the past 20 years, I've helped thousands of clients realize and appreciate the healing properties of massage. This experience ignited my passion for natural wellness, and sustains it to this day. Share with me in that enthusiasm as we discover what other cultures throughout the world have known for generations.

Long thought to be a luxury reserved for celebrities and spa junkies, massage therapy began to achieve mass appeal in the United States toward the end of the 20th century, coinciding with a growing interest in natural wellness. From airport kiosks to mobile massage, this therapy has never been more accessible.

Though massage didn't make its way to the U.S. until the mid-1800s, the practice itself dates back thousands of years to ancient India, where it was—and still is—a major part of the "life medicine" practice known as Ayurveda.

Massage made its way to Asia around 2700 BC, where practitioners of Chinese medicine incorporated into it elements of martial arts and yoga. Today, those methods also include acupuncture and acupressure.

Ancient Egyptian paintings contain representations of massage being performed, and it is thought that the technique known as reflexology originated during this period. Around 1000 BC, Buddhist monks introduced massage therapy to the Japanese, who developed the shiatsu modality. Later, the Egyptians brought massage to the Greeks and Romans, who used it with athletes in preparation for competition. Advances in modern medicine led to a decline in the popularity of massage therapy until it was "rediscovered" by Swedish doctor Per Ling, who developed a technique thought to be the forebearer of the modern Swedish massage. The Dutch doctor Johan Mezger added five specific strokes to Ling's version, all of which are currently used today.

Massage therapy made its way to North America from Europe during the 19th century, when it was combined with other spa services, such as exfoliation and facial masks. Massage gained legitimacy in the 1930s when it became used more regularly in medical practices. Soon, though, the practice was pushed to the side by the excitement of a burgeoning pharmaceutical industry. Within decades, however, shifting attitudes on fitness, diet, and healthy living would make *wellness* an everyday word. And that's where we find ourselves today. Alternative therapies are no longer so alternative, and proponents of this approach don't find themselves so much at odds with the medical establishment. On the contrary, that once-antagonistic relationship has been supplanted by a shared focus on prevention, as evidenced by the many premier medical institutions that now have dedicated integrative health departments. Massage therapy is among many natural wellness strategies now being recommended by conventionally trained physicians.

TYPES OF MASSAGE

Massage is for everyone! Through their training, licensed massage therapists have gained a thorough understanding of the musculoskeletal system. During an initial visit, your provider will perform an assessment which, along with your feedback, will form the basis of a customized treatment plan. There are more than 75 types of massage, and modalities are often combined for best results. These are among the most commonly used:

SWEDISH

The most popular type of massage, Swedish is based on five specific strokes, long and flowing in nature: effleurage, petrissage, friction, vibration, and tapotement. This full-body technique involves mild pressure and kneading of the muscles. Swedish massage is best suited for those with surface-level tension and anyone looking for a state of general relaxation.

DEEP TISSUE

Deep tissue incorporates the same strokes as in Swedish massage, but the therapist makes use of the elbows and forearms to apply additional pressure. More attention will be directed to trouble spots, or "knots," at the direction of the client. Deep tissue is particularly effective for those who engage regularly in strenuous exercise or those with certain types of injuries, such as disc issues.

SPORTS

As the name would imply, a sports massage is intended to help with recovery from athletic endeavors. This type of massage is similar to deep tissue but typically involves various stretches, and may be more targeted to address areas of the body that are particularly stiff or sore. It's also a more vigorous massage. Increased range of motion is one of the many benefits you can expect from a sports massage.

TRIGGER POINT

A trigger point is a tight spot, or knot, in the muscle. Often caused by overuse, these tender, sensitive areas can sometimes impinge on nerves, causing tingling and numbness in other areas of the body. This is known as "referred pain." Trigger-point massage utilizes the fingertips and other tools, applying direct pressure on the knot for a period of at least several minutes.

THAI

Unlike other types of massage, there are no oils or lotions used in traditional Thai massage, and the client remains fully clothed. Thai massage borrows from yoga practice and incorporates a variety of stretches, poses, and postures. Though it may be relaxing for some, the aim is more therapeutic.

SHIATSU

Having originated in Japan and based on Chinese medicine, shiatsu massage targets specific energy "paths" in the body similar to acupuncture. This modality is also performed fully clothed.

HOT STONE

The warmth and weight of these smooth, basalt stones helps to loosen the muscles. This makes it easier for the therapist to access the muscles and to apply deeper pressure.

REFLEXOLOGY

This modality targets nerve endings in the hands, ears, and feet that correspond to other parts of the body, including internal organs. Reflexology aims to restore the flow of energy throughout the body.

CRANIOSACRAL

If you know your anatomy, you understand that this type of massage targets the skull, spinal column, and pelvic region. This therapy focuses on bones and not just muscles.

This isn't an exhaustive list. There's also sleep massage, facial massage, CBD massage, abdominal massage, lymphatic drainage, and myofascial release. Sometimes, massage is combined with related methods, such as rolfing and cupping, or other alternative treatments like aromatherapy.

We no longer seek massage simply to *feel* better; we get massages to live better. According to a survey by the American Massage Therapy Association, 75% of respondents indicate that their main reason for getting a massage over the past year was medical.

In just the last decade, considerable research has accumulated to confirm what those of us in the profession—along with our clients—have always known: The benefits of massage therapy are numerous, and extend far beyond the obvious. While the evidence is stronger in some areas than in others and though additional studies will be needed to further advance our understanding, a consensus has formed that the effects of massage on a range of health issues are more than just anecdotal. Here is a sampling of those scientific findings.

STRESS AND ANXIETY

* Muscles tighten when we're feeling stressed. Massage helps to eliminate that tension and induce a state of calm.

* Research conducted at the Mood and Anxiety Disorders Program of Emory University found that massage greatly improves symptoms of generalized anxiety based on Hamilton Anxiety Rating Scale (HARS) scores.

* A review in the *International Journal of Neuroscience* concluded that massage improves emotional resilience and well-being.

* Indirectly, massage can help with other issues related to psychological stress, including focus and concentration, and even digestion.

DEPRESSION

* Because massage therapy takes place in a secure, caring environment and a trusting relationship can be built with the practitioner over time, massage is thought to help those with depression.

ASTHMA

* When used in conjunction with conventional treatment, craniosacral massage may improve asthma symptoms according to one study.

FIBROMYALGIA

* Based on research in this area, massage can provide immediate improvements in the pain and anxiety associated with fibromyalgia.

CHRONIC FATIGUE SYNDROME (CFS)

* This condition, that causes pain in the muscles and tendons, has no known cause. Chronic Fatigue Syndrome affects more than one million Americans. Massage has been found to help with some of the symptoms of CFS—such as anxiety and sleep dysfunction—which can overlap with those of fibromyalgia.

MULTIPLE SCLEROSIS (MS)

* A 2009 study suggested that craniosacral therapy could relieve some of the urinary tract symptoms common among MS patients.

SKIN

* The impact of our stressful lives is reflected in our skin. Massage helps to rid the body of dead skin, improves circulation (which stimulates regeneration of the cells), expands blood vessels (which improves our complexion), and may even make scars less visible.

INSOMNIA

* In a 2011 Brazilian study using Sleep Diary, researchers found that "all participants fell asleep faster, experienced improved quality of sleep and felt better upon waking."

JOINTS

* Not only is massage considered safe for those with arthritis, but a study published in the *Journal of General Internal Medicine* in 2018 noted dramatic improvement in mobility among individuals with knee osteoarthritis who received a one-hour weekly massage.

* Additional research from a study at the University of Miami found that a 15-minute daily massage could improve grip strength in those with arthritis of the hands and wrists. Results from the same study suggested an improvement in hand pain of up to 57%.

PAIN

* This is one of the biggest reasons people seek out massage. Research supports its effectiveness in this area. Massage can reduce soreness, for example, by 30% in just 10 minutes according to one study.

* Lower-back pain is one of the most common ailments suffered by Americans. Research has indicated an important role for massage in addressing this issue.

TMJ

* Massage of the muscles in the area around the temporomandibular joint can alleviate the jaw pain and stiffness associated with TMJ, which is commonly caused by clenching the teeth.

HEADACHES

* Research has shown that massage can lessen the pain caused by migraine headaches.

* A 2002 study published in the *American Journal of Public Health* demonstrated "a significant and meaningful reduction" in the "frequency and duration" of tension headaches.

JUVENILE RHEUMATOID ARTHRITIS

* Research has shown an immediate decrease in pain and anxiety among test subjects suffering from this autoimmune disease.

CANCER-RELATED FATIGUE

* Swedish massage led to a "significant reduction" in cancer-related fatigue (CRF) according to one study.

MITOCHONDRIAL BIOGENESIS

* You may recall from your high-school biology class that these cellular "powerhouses" are responsible for turning the food we eat into energy. Mitochondrial biogenesis refers to the production of new mitochondria, a process that is triggered by regular exercise, but also through massage therapy. We typically lose mitochondria as we age, and this has been implicated in the development of chronic disease. Increasing mitochondria is thought to slow this process.

IMMUNE FUNCTION

* According to researchers at Cedars-Sinai Medical Center in Los Angeles, massage helps boost the production of lymphocytes and reduces levels of inflammatory molecules called cytokines.

* Additional research has found that massage increases levels of tumor-destroying natural "killer" T cells.

* Reflexology can favorably alter the balance of our T-helper 1 (Th1) and T-helper 2 (Th2) cells, according to a 2010 study in *Experimental and therapeutic medicine*. These immune cells have specialized roles in fighting cancer and extracellular pathogens, respectively.

Massage therapy exerts its benefits through several mechanisms.

1. MECHANICAL PRESSURE

In simple terms, massage is the physical manipulation of the soft tissue by means of direct pressure. This triggers various responses within the body:

* Realignment of soft tissue

This one is fairly obvious. The prolonged sitting that defines modern life takes a serious toll on the body that goes beyond weight management considerations. Sitting causes muscle imbalances, spinal misalignment, postural issues, and wear and tear on our discs. When muscle fibers stick together, a knot, or adhesion, forms. Not only do tight muscles restrict movement, they can also impact nerve signaling to the brain.

The manipulation of soft tissue by a massage therapist can help to correct some of these issues by breaking down and realigning the muscle fibers. In addition, massage can calm the muscle spasms that occur with overexertion.

* Increased circulation of blood and lymph

The friction created by the therapist's hands warms the muscles and stimulates the process of vasodilation, or the widening of blood vessels. This allows for enhanced delivery of oxygen and nutrients to damaged muscles and joints, speeding up the healing process.

The lymphatic system is activated by muscular contraction. This pumps lymphatic fluid (and the metabolic waste it contains) through the body for removal. However, this process is hindered when the muscles are tight, allowing toxins to accumulate. The mechanical pressure of massage therapy helps to get the lymph moving again. The same process also helps reduce swelling.

2. RELAXATION

Most of us associate massage with relaxation but how exactly is this achieved? There are several processes involved:

* Neurotransmitters

These are brain chemicals released into the bloodstream during massage. They include endorphins, oxytocin, dopamine, and serotonin. By countering the action of stress hormones like cortisol, these neurotransmitters enhance mood and create feelings of positivity. In that sense, massage changes our biochemistry, with one study showing a 31% reduction in cortisol and norepinephrine, with a simultaneous 30% increase in the "pleasure" hormones dopamine and serotonin.

* Other effects on the nervous system

When our nerve receptors sense physical touch, they send signals to the brain, which turn on the parasympathetic nervous system. This results in a slowing of the heart rate and a relaxing of other organs and bodily functions. It also counters the effects of the sympathetic nervous system, which leaves us in a perpetual state of "fight-or-flight." You'll learn elsewhere in the book how short-term, or acute, stress is an evolutionary adaptation that can be beneficial in small doses. Chronic physical and psychological stress, on the other hand, increases anxiety and inflammation. Besides massage, many additional modalities and other lifestyle modifications can help us to balance our sympathetic and parasympathetic responses. We'll discuss those in the next chapter.

Much of this activity is controlled by the vagus nerve, which connects the brain with other parts of the body, such as the gut. Vagal activity impacts heart rate, breathing, and digestion, among other processes. Increased vagal tone is linked to enhanced parasympathetic response. Many of the stress-relieving benefits of massage therapy are due to its ability to improve vagal tone, as this is associated with higher levels of mood-boosting dopamine and serotonin. This is also the mechanism through which deep breathing, meditation, and laughter help with relaxation. Targeting specific areas of the body with massage, and through reflexology specifically, has been shown to increase vagal tone.

3. INFLAMMATION

Exercise-induced muscle pain and soreness results from a process called microtrauma, in which muscle fibers sustain tears. This triggers an inflammatory response by the body as a means of healing the damaged tissue. Research has shown that massage therapy can speed up the recovery process after a bout of exercise by decreasing levels of inflammation. The mechanism is similar to that of non-steroidal anti-inflammatory drugs (NSAIDs), but without the side effects.

* As in any other profession, an unqualified provider can do more harm than good. The best way to go about finding a reputable and skilled massage therapist is to seek a referral from a friend, your doctor, a personal trainer, physical therapist, or chiropractor. The American Massage Therapy Association and the National Certification Board for Therapeutic Massage & Bodywork are also trusted resources for locating a provider.

* In terms of frequency, most of the research in this area has found benefits when massage is performed at least once weekly.

* Communication with your provider is crucial. Massage therapists are trained in many modalities and can make use of a range of pressure levels and strategies based on your lifestyle, injury status, medical history, and comfort level. Don't be shy!

> " Anyone wishing to study medicine must master the art of massage. "
>
> - Hippocrates, the father of modern medicine

Now you can see why more and more Americans are seeking massage as their first choice of alternative therapies. Tight, stiff, and sore is no way to go through life, but as you've discovered, the benefits of massage go far beyond a more fluid body. Hippocrates knew that all the way back in the 5th century. What else can we learn from these ancient schools of medicine? Keep reading and discover that what's old is new again.

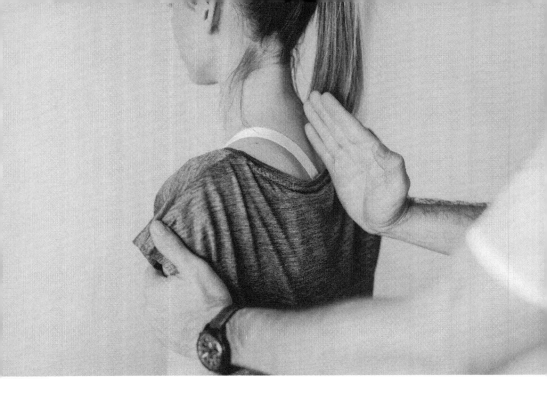

CHAPTER 06

Other Therapies—Chiropractic, Acupuncture, Reiki, Hypnosis, Naturopathy

It's never been a more exciting time to be a student or practitioner of natural wellness. The field has come so far that it's even been given an acronym. Complementary and alternative medicine, or CAM, encompasses the body manipulation therapies we discussed in the previous chapter, natural products such as dietary supplements, our focus in Chapter 8 and so much more.

Massage is one of the most commonly used CAM practices and, but in this section, we'll highlight several other popular therapies. First, though, let's take a few minutes to appreciate the breadth and depth of what we're talking about.

Though the terms are sometimes used interchangeably, it's important to distinguish between alternative and complementary medicine. While alternative therapies are meant to be used *instead* of the traditional Western, or allopathic, approach, complementary therapies are incorporated *alongside* standard medical practice. The two together are part of the broader field of integrative medicine, a holistic approach to healthcare now embraced by distinguished institutions such as Duke, Yale, Johns Hopkins, and the Cleveland Clinic.

The rapid growth in this area stems, in part, from an increased awareness of the limitations and failings of modern medicine. The news media report on a declining life expectancy and a chronic health crisis in the U.S., which only confirms what we experience each day—firsthand with our own bodies, while caring for a loved one, or when walking down the street.

Perhaps we've hit our collective rock bottom, but it can also be said that we've begun a slow but steady upward trajectory. Nearly half of all Americans use at least one form of complementary and alternative medicine, and 70 percent of respondents in one survey say they have a favorable view of CAM. The list of available options continues to grow, but three of the most popular treatments are chiropractic, acupuncture, reiki, and hypnosis.

CHIROPRACTIC

Chiropractors were once thought of as nothing more than "bone crackers" and dismissed as charlatans. Fast-forward to 2020 and the treatment they offer is now recommended by the American College of Physicians for managing acute lower back pain—the type you incur when moving a couch, for example. Evidence for chiropractic care also supports its use in treating neck and shoulder pain, as well as athletic injuries.

Chiropractors are trained in the identification and treatment of neuromusculoskeletal disorders and can also assess misalignment of the spine and other structural imbalances. Though chiropractic care is most often associated with spinal manipulation, a treatment session may also include ergonomic education, exercise instruction, and postural analysis and correction.

Like massage therapy, chiropractic exerts its benefits, in part, by triggering the release of endorphins. Recall from the previous chapter that these pain-fighting, pleasure-boosting, opioid-like chemicals are released by the pituitary gland in response to physical or psychological stress. As with other healing methods that rely on touch, chiropractic treatments also enhance circulation and improve range of motion.

Today's chiropractors use a range of methods. Manual release therapy is the most basic, and involves stretching a muscle while simultaneously applying pressure. As we highlighted in the previous chapter, trigger-point therapy uses direct and more prolonged pressure on muscles that are particularly tense.

Some chiropractors perform soft tissue therapy using tools or instruments, including a transcutaneous electrical nerve stimulator (TENS), which delivers an electric current to targeted regions of the body. This warms the surface of the skin, increases circulation, quiets the body's pain signals, and activates the endorphin system. Research has shown that TENS therapy is effective in reducing pain caused by conditions such as fibromyalgia. While TENS works on nerve pathways, electric muscle stimulation (EMS) is used to treat muscle spasms and inflammation, and is more often seen in athletic training or a rehabilitation setting.

Whether used on their own or in combination, these noninvasive therapies can often eliminate the need for surgery, saving us money down the road. There's also no downtime associated with chiropractic care.

Despite myths to the contrary, chiropractic adjustments are rarely painful and a lifelong commitment is not necessary. We're hard on our bodies, though, and if you're part of the majority of Americans who sit for eight hours a day, you might benefit from regular visits. A qualified chiropractor can help you learn more about how your body moves and can provide self-care tips to help you maintain it over the long-term.

Rooted in traditional Chinese medicine, acupuncture is centered around the belief that disease results from an obstructed flow of energy, or Qi. The treatment involves the strategic placement of very thin needles into *acupoints*. These are inserted anywhere between 1⁄4 to one inch deep, depending on the condition being addressed.

While acupuncture is most commonly used to manage pain and symptoms of stress, research sponsored by the National Institutes of Health (NIH) has shown that acupuncture is an effective treatment alone or in combination with conventional therapies to address the following:

- Nausea caused by surgical anesthesia and cancer chemotherapy

- Dental pain after surgery

- Addiction

- Headaches

- Menstrual cramps

- Tennis elbow

- Fibromyalgia

- Osteoarthritis

- Carpal tunnel syndrome

- Asthma

- Stroke rehabilitation

An analysis of nearly two dozen studies demonstrated the effectiveness of acupuncture in treating low back pain. A 2017 review in the *Journal of Pain* found that acupuncture is beneficial for those suffering from chronic pain and that the effects are lasting. Additional research has suggested that acupuncture can make weight-loss methods more effective when combined.

As the quality of the research improves, it becomes clear that the benefits of acupuncture can no longer be attributed to placebo. In comparison to exercise and weight loss, acupuncture was found in one study to be more effective as a treatment for knee osteoarthritis.

In research on shoulder impingement syndrome, acupuncture outperformed steroid injection, NSAIDs, ultrasound, and nearly a dozen other treatment options. And a 2016 review of 20 interventions found acupuncture to be the second most effective for treating sciatica, besting drugs, exercise, and surgery.

We're not totally sure why acupuncture works as well as it does, but we do know that, like massage and chiropractic, acupuncture can stimulate endorphin release and exerts anti-inflammatory and immune-boosting effects.

Responses vary by individual, with some experiencing a sense of calm afterwards and others finding themselves more stimulated. This may be due to the use of different styles of acupuncture. Some practitioners, for example, will incorporate heat during the treatment; others use a form of suction known as cupping.

Regardless of the method, acupuncture is considered safe, with only a mild ache or stinging being reported at the insertion site. This sensation is considered a sign that the needle has hit its intended target and that the treatment is exerting a benefit.

Reiki, sometimes referred to as energy healing, is a form of alternative medicine that originated in Japan. Similar to some other therapies we've discussed, reiki is based on the concept that weak, inhibited, or imbalanced energy within the body can cause physical and emotional symptoms.

Reiki treatment takes place in a quiet, comfortable setting and involves the placement of the practitioner's hands on or just above the patient's fully clothed body. Starting with the head, the reiki master redirects the flow of energy to activate the body's natural healing abilities. The practitioner's hands are held in one position until it is determined that the energy has diminished.

While various techniques may be employed, reiki requires no specialized equipment and can be performed anywhere. The length of a reiki session will vary based on one's goals, with the average duration between 30 and 60 minutes.

Hundreds of hospitals in the U.S. now offer reiki as a complementary treatment in patients suffering anxiety, depression, and fatigue. A 2006 study found that reiki can lower stress levels in women scheduled for hysterectomies, and more recent research has demonstrated a similar effect in cancer patients. Evidence also supports the use of reiki as a way to improve well-being and relieve pain. Anecdotally, patients report feeling more relaxed after a reiki session and many say they gain a sense of mental clarity from the treatment.

HYPNOSIS

Hundreds of years after it was first used in the U.S., hypnotherapy remains shrouded in mystery. Like many of the other treatments we've discussed, it has been surrounded by myths and misconceptions, mostly due to how the practice has been depicted in pop culture.

As it turns out, though, hypnosis is useful for more than just unearthing long-buried memories. It's been studied extensively and has now gained mainstream acceptance as a complementary treatment for a growing list of mental and physical health issues.

When combined with other forms of psychotherapy, such as cognitive-behavioral therapy (CBT), hypnosis leads to greater weight loss and less regain than with CBT on its own. Hypnosis has also been shown to reduce post-operative pain in children and in a 2008 study at Yale-New Haven Hospital, hypnosis alleviated pain and anxiety among kids receiving intravenous lines in the emergency room.

In a separate study, hypnotherapy helped ease stress and discomfort in adults undergoing treatment for irritable bowel syndrome (IBS). It's also been found to make epidural work significantly more effective for managing pain during labor and delivery.

Hypnosis has become recognized as an effective addition to many smoking cessation programs, having been shown to work better than standard therapy in helping smokers to quit their habit. Hypnotherapy has even demonstrated the ability to boost immunity and fight off viral infections.

While there's no clear-cut explanation as to how the process exerts its many benefits, a typical hypnosis session involves two distinct phases. During *induction*, the patient enters a relaxed state, quiets their thoughts, and centers their attention on the therapist. This can happen in a matter of seconds; it may also require several minutes. In the *suggestion* phase, the therapist takes the patient through imaginary scenarios, introducing cues that will help them in similar situation when the trance is complete.

Hypnosis targets various parts of the brain, including those associated with the pain response and the processing of emotions. While the idea of an altered state might spook you, the trance is what makes us more open to suggestion. This gives us the control to overcome any blocks we encounter in problematic situations.

Some individuals are less receptive to induction than others. Treatment almost always requires more than one session. It's important to note that hypnosis is just one of many psychotherapeutic techniques.

Often used interchangeably, the terms *integrative, holistic,* and *naturopathic* all refer to the use of a combination of both modern and traditional forms of medicine to bring the body into a state of balance and trigger its natural healing powers. The naturopathic umbrella covers diet and nutrition, physical activity, stress reduction, herbalism, and social wellness, among several other facets. Many of these ancient practices have been proven effective through scientific research and some of the plant-based therapies have even formed the basis of the pharmaceutical treatments that define allopathic medicine.

A naturopathic physician is typically trained in a four or five year post graduate program that requires more than 1,200 hours of supervised clinical training and over 300 credit hours of biomedical science instruction, which includes conventional pharmacology. They take national licensing exams similar to conventional medical boards. Naturopathic schools are accredited by the federal government. Naturopathic doctors are trained as primary care physicians, and practice as such in many states.

Naturopathic physicians are regarded as much for their listening skills as they are for their ability to heal. Armed with a thorough understanding of the patient as an individual, the naturopathic physician is better equipped to identify root causes of illness and to design customized treatment plans accordingly.

- These treatments are considered safe when performed by a trained, licensed practitioner. In addition to recommendations from friends and family, refer to these professional organizations for help with finding a qualified provider:

    1. American Chiropractic Association

    2. International Chiropractors Association

    3. National Certification Commission for Acupuncture and Oriental Medicine

    4. American Society of Acupuncturists

    5. Center for Reiki Research

    6. International Association of Reiki Professionals

    7. National Board of Certified Clinical Hypnotherapists

- Benefits from CAM tend to be cumulative, so be patient. Your first few sessions may seem uneventful, but that doesn't mean the therapy hasn't had an effect on a cellular, metabolic, or hormonal level.

- Let your provider know about any shyness you may have about being touched. If you are pregnant or undergoing medical treatment or if certain body positions cause discomfort or trouble breathing, communicate those as well.

- Aetna, Anthem, Blue Cross and many other insurance companies now cover at least some of the cost of many CAM treatments.

- This represents only a sampling of the available CAM therapies. Evidence is mounting in support of other treatments, including music therapy, and botanical, or herbal, medicine. Speak with a CAM-savvy physician to determine the best treatment plan for you.

Skeptics of CAM often conflate the terms "unproven" and "disproven" to argue that such therapies are ineffective or unsafe. But few scientific theories are ever disproven (it's hard to prove a negative) and, in the absence of clinical trials, other evidence is available with which to make reasonable assessments.

The naysayers also fail to acknowledge some of the methodological challenges involved in testing CAM treatments. And while many of us assume that the therapies used in modern medicine have been rigorously tested, that is not always the case. Aside from being expensive, conventional treatments can carry with them the risk of serious adverse effects. Is the science behind CAM definitive? No, but we routinely prescribe drugs like opioids, a practice that has contributed to a public health crisis. And doctors don't wait for ironclad evidence before recommending an off-label use of certain medications. These issues are not black and white, and the patient suffers when the discussion is framed that way.

While CAM might not be for everyone and though the most firmly entrenched doubters will always be distrustful of these methods, Ayurvedic and traditional Chinese medicine have been practiced for thousands of years—and continue to this day—in parts of the world with much lower disease rates than we experience here in the U.S.

We do emergency medicine really well in this country, better than anyplace else in the world. But we fail miserably when it comes to prevention, and it's clear that what we've been doing to fight chronic disease hasn't been effective. Americans are demanding more from mainstream medicine, and any discussion of healthcare reform in this country should include a thorough consideration of this reality.

The use of multiple strategies in the prevention and treatment of disease improves outcomes. Having more weapons in our wellness arsenal can also help reduce healthcare costs. This type of broader, more coordinated care puts the patient in control and the whole-person approach makes conventional medicine work better.

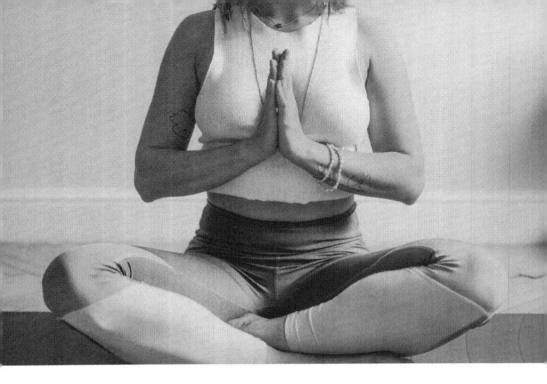

CHAPTER 07

Relax, Meditate

There was a time when an anxiety attack was considered little more than a temporary distraction. Sweaty palms and a racing heart? How about a stiff drink to take the edge off? Pop some Alka-Seltzer to ease your nervous stomach and you'd be ready to face the world again.

Our understanding of stress and anxiety has evolved quite a bit from the days of mother's little helper. While these issues were assumed to be "all in our heads," we now know that psychological stress triggers a cascade of events within the body that can shorten our lives.

According to a recent review, "the overall data suggest that stress contributes to adverse clinical cardiac events and provides a milieu of increased vulnerability to the heart."

Scientists are not suggesting that stress *causes* heart disease, but it's become increasingly clear in recent years that chronic stress can contribute to known risk factors for atherosclerosis. Higher levels of hormones such as adrenaline and cortisol, for example, cause increases in blood sugar, blood pressure, cholesterol, and triglycerides. Stress also triggers inflammation, which can lead to plaque accumulation. In fact, studies on individuals who have experienced trauma have found blocked arteries and other damage to the heart muscle.

One study examined the effects of stress among females going through divorce. Researchers found that these women had an increased risk of heart attack on par with that of a smoker or someone with diabetes!

Job stress can affect your heart as well. Based on one study, if you're worried about losing your job, your chance of developing heart disease goes up about 20 percent.

Part of this effect may be indirect. Stressed individuals are more likely to engage in behaviors linked to an increased risk of heart disease: drug and alcohol abuse, smoking, physical inactivity, and poor diet.

Then there's the phenomenon of *broken heart syndrome*. Its official name is takotsubo cardiomyopathy, a condition in which the left ventricle of the heart becomes damaged in response to a stressful event such as the loss of a loved one.

Chronic stress can also suppress immunity. Specifically, it can decrease levels of white blood cells and natural killer (NK) cells. This leaves us more prone to viral infections and can trigger the growth of tumors.

In research on students studying for an exam—a simple stressor—it was found that the participants' bodies nearly stopped making immunity-boosting gamma interferon and that the response of their T-cells toward a stimulated infection was weakened. The students had been shown relaxation techniques beforehand. Those who neglected that training had worse outcomes; the students who more strictly adhered to relaxation protocols experienced "significantly" better immune response during exams.

Research reveals that elderly individuals or those with preexisting health issues fare worse when it comes to stress-related immune dysfunction. In this case, even mild depression might lower immunity in an older adult, and in one study, T-cell response to foreign invaders was still weak more than one year later! These results are consistent with previous research demonstrating that the duration of a mental illness—in this case, depression—is a more significant factor in stress-related immune change than is the severity of the condition.

——— **QUICK FIX OR ROOT CAUSE?**

In 2017, the American Psychological Association announced that Americans are more stressed than ever before. And things have only gotten worse since then. We're stressed about the path we're taking as a country. We're stressed about our jobs and the economy, our health, our relationships.

- According to a 2020 Gallup poll, more than 60% of Americans report being stressed every day.

- A survey by Everest College found that 83% of us feel stressed at work and Dynamic Signal reported that 63% of Americans would like to quit their jobs because of it.

- Research conducted by Everyday Health found that one-third of Americans sought medical treatment in 2018 for stress-related symptoms. The same group found that—for those who experience stress—57% say they are "paralyzed" by it.

The effects of stress are cumulative, but they are also modifiable through behavior change. Unfortunately, an increasing number of Americans are deciding it's easier to numb themselves with benzodiazepines, such as Xanax. More than one-fourth of doctor's visits in this country result in a prescription for a benzodiazepine, and their use has tripled since 1995. These antianxiety drugs are intended to be used for short periods of time, but more of us are getting hooked, an issue that some experts are beginning to equate to the opioid epidemic. A class of antidepressants known as selective serotonin uptake inhibitors (SSRIs) is thought to be less habit-forming, but side effects can include *increased* anxiety and sexual dysfunction and the withdrawal symptoms from these drugs can last more than a year.

I've discussed many other drug-free stress reduction modalities in this book, but meditation is one of the oldest and most effective and is worthy of a more thorough review.

WHAT IS MEDITATION?

Think of it as exercise for the mind. The *muscle* you're working is called resilience, a form of mental toughness that becomes a coping mechanism in the face of adversity.

Rooted in ancient Buddhist tradition, meditation gives us the strength to break free from situations over which we have no control. Modern-day practitioners refer to this as being *present*.

WHY MEDITATION?

Most individuals who begin a meditation program do so for stress relief. Psychotherapy and antidepressants don't always help. For some patients, they don't help at all. Meditation provides an alternative for those non-responders and can be used on its own, or in combination with more conventional treatments. Research from the David Lynch Foundation reveals that meditation can decrease the symptoms of emotional distress by 40%.

Meditation works its magic through several pathways but its most powerful effects stem from its ability to shrink the amygdala over time. This part of the brain processes some of our most unpleasant emotions. So meditation literally changes your brain. This is called neuroplasticity and it allows nerve cells to strengthen themselves and to adapt to new stimuli. Functional magnetic resonance imaging (fMRI) scans have also shown that meditation can increase the size of the hippocampus. This region of the brain is responsible for memory and learning.

THE BENEFITS OF MEDITATION

* Stress reduction

* Inner peace

* A sense of calm

* New coping skills

- Acceptance

- Better sleep

- Patience

- Positive attitude

- More creativity

- Mental sharpness

Perhaps the biggest benefit is that anyone can do it—anywhere—and safely.

WHAT DOES THE SCIENCE SAY?

Hundreds of studies have looked into the health benefits of meditation. Here is just a sampling of those results.

1. A 2016 article published in *NeuroImage* found that meditation slows brain aging. Researchers determined that the brains of meditators were 7.5 years younger than those of the control group.

2. A 2012 study demonstrated that meditation can improve focus and problem-solving.

3. A 2018 Harvard University study found that an eight-week meditation program favorably altered the expression of genes involved in inflammation, circadian rhythm, and glucose metabolism. This resulted in reduced blood pressure readings.

4. A 2012 study found that meditation blunts stress-induced inflammation and increases activity in areas of the brain that help us to adapt and remain calm in the face of stress.

5. Research published in 2013 in *Psychological Science* reported that meditation makes us more caring and compassionate in response to others' suffering.

6. Meditation can improve the symptoms of fibromyalgia.

7. Meditation can enhance mood and fight stress in cancer patients.

8. A 2008 study in the Journal of Behavioral Medicine showed that an eight-week meditation program was able to improve symptoms of anxiety, obsessive-compulsive disorder, and paranoia.

9. Research has demonstrated that meditation is effective in treating insomnia.

10. Participants in a smoking-cessation program were several times more successful in kicking the habit after meditation training than those who relied on a more traditional program developed by the American Lung Association.

Other health issues that may benefit from regular meditation include irritable bowel syndrome (IBS), pain disorders, and certain types of headaches. Researchers at the University of Wisconsin at Madison even reported that the flu vaccine is more effective in meditators.

TYPES OF MEDITATION

Meditation is a broad term and encompasses various methods of stress reduction. What these all have in common is the "relaxation response," a physical state first described in the 1970s by Harvard University professor Herbert Benson. He characterized it as the opposite of our fight-or-flight reaction, which is a survival response regulated by the sympathetic nervous system. The resulting increase in alertness, heart rate, blood pressure, and adrenaline served our paleolithic ancestors well when being chased by a lion, but these days *threats* are more often in the form of a traffic jam or a work deadline. Our frenetic modern existence finds us spending much of our days stuck in a sympathetic state. Meditation and other mindfulness techniques turn on the parasympathetic nervous system and return us to a more relaxed state.

- **Mindfulness meditation** - a focus on breath and environment

- **Guided meditation** - also called guided imagery; led by a teacher who walks you through the inner workings of the mind

- **Transcendental meditation** - a "resting practice" that focuses on a chosen mantra and is most often taught by an instructor

- **Metta meditation** - an "outward" form of meditation in which we give well-wishes and expressions of love and kindness to others

- **Chakra meditation** - a focus on opening the body's seven "energy centers," or chakras

- **Vipassana meditation** - teaches deep awareness of physical sensations (itching, tingling, pressure) and our reactions to them

As a means of looking inward, meditation is closely related to prayer. Practices such as yoga, tai chi, and qigong are forms of *moving* meditation.

1. LOSE THE STEREOTYPES

No, meditation is not just for "new-age hippy types." You don't have to become a vegan and you don't need to wear special clothes. Likewise, meditation doesn't require sitting cross-legged in a dark, quiet room. If you've been clinging to these myths, maybe you're actually just afraid of your own thoughts!

2. DROP THE EXCUSES

Don't have time to meditate? Start with five minutes, it's better than nothing (the Aura app has meditations as short as three minutes).Your goal should be to build up to 20 minutes. If you've bought into the need for it and are convinced of the benefits, it shouldn't be hard to motivate yourself. Block off the time in your daily schedule, just as you would a trip to the gym. Once you begin to reap some benefits, you'll likely be hooked and you'll find yourself making more time for it. It's that powerful!

3. PAY CLOSE ATTENTION TO YOUR PRE-MEDITATION RITUAL

Stimulating activities can make it much harder to achieve the necessary focus, calm, and relaxation. Cut out the following at least one hour before meditating:

- Processed foods or those high in sugar

- Coffee or other sources of caffeine

- Television, movies, or video games, particularly those of an intense nature

- Computers, phones, email, social media

Instead, take a bath or shower, perform light stretches, listen to some soothing music, or read a book.

4. START WITH GUIDED MEDITATION

Sometimes referred to as guided imagery or visualization, this is a good option for beginners. Your goal, however, is to progress to silent meditation. Guided meditation involves narration (and often music), which can be distracting and can prevent access to your inner thoughts.

5. CONSIDER AN APP

Calm and Headspace are two of the most popular. Headspace is more structured, user-friendly, and has more options for beginners. Calm has features that may appeal more to experienced meditators. Both offer a free trial; a one-year subscription is about $70.

6. USE A TIMER

Wondering how long you've been sitting in silence can make some folks restless. A timer can be set to alert you at periodic intervals throughout and at the end of your meditation session. Beginners may choose to schedule short breaks to make a longer session seem less daunting. This can also help you stay grounded if your mind tends to wander. Timers are a great way to track your progress as well. Insight Timer is the most popular and there are many others.

7. OTHER RESOURCES

I recommend *The Mind Illuminated* by John Yates, Matthew Immergut, and Jeremy Graves. This is a thorough, science-based, practical guide. Podcasts have helped make the practice of meditation more mainstream. Some of the best meditation podcasts are: Ten Percent Happier, Untangle, Tara Brach, and the OneMind Podcast. The streaming music service Spotify offers a wide range of meditation playlists and YouTube has no shortage of videos for meditators of all experience levels.

8. DON'T OVERCOMPLICATE IT

We hear a lot about the importance of breathing in meditation, but the breath is intended only as a focal point to which we return when our mind drifts. The breath is automatic—it's always there—and feeling and hearing it helps us practice awareness. There are other ways to achieve this, however. Some meditators choose to concentrate on the flame of a candle, for example. Others prefer to repeat a mantra anytime they begin to lose focus. This can be any positive and uplifting word or phrase. Meditation can also be an opportunity for reflection. Think back on your day, your week, your life. What are you grateful for? Do it your way. The only rule is this: no self-judgement!

Skeptics are understandably intimidated (and, perhaps, turned off) when proponents of mindfulness practice talk of things like "retraining subconscious awareness." To the uninitiated, abstract concepts like *journey* and *purpose* are also pie-in-the-sky. Let's keep it simple.

In the words of Indian meditation and spiritual master, Sadhguru:

> 66 Life has no purpose—and that's the great thing about it. You can always discover new things. If there is something like a purpose for humans, you finish it and life would have no meaning from this point on. 99

One might also say that the purpose is to create your own purpose. And if you don't want to have a purpose then that's your purpose. Perhaps your purpose is to be free from inner conflict and self-judgement. Meditation can help with that, and the benefits extend well beyond the session. You'll be able to calm yourself faster and more effectively in stressful situations. Your breathing will become deeper. You'll be less impulsive. You'll have a brighter outlook. You may even find that your memory improves. Anxiety is a result of expectations you have for yourself that you fear you cannot meet. Meditation takes away the expectations and the fear. And it just may extend your life.

Need more inspiration? Here's a list of some pretty successful people who meditate. You may recognize a few of their names:

* Oprah Winfrey

* Katy Perry

* Madonna

* Jennifer Lopez

* Paul McCartney

* Jerry Seinfeld

* Bill Gates

* Jeff Weiner, CEO of LinkedIn

* William Clay Ford, Jr., Executive Chairman of Ford Motor Company

Pretty good company, eh?

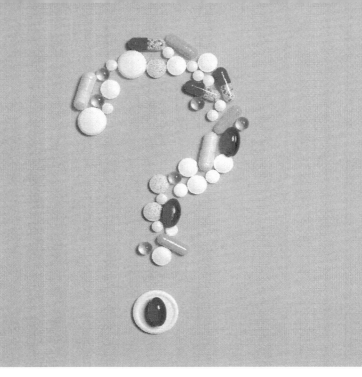

CHAPTER 08

Why Supplements?
Junk Science vs. Real Science

Confused about supplements? You're not alone. Like so many other issues these days, the decision to take dietary supplements has become somewhat polarized, with *pro* and *anti* camps having emerged. The conversation has been framed as an either-or proposition, leading many of us to feel we need to pick a side.

But when it comes to our health, there shouldn't be *sides*. We should be guided by a thorough review of *all* available evidence, free from sensationalism and hype. Health news writers in this country have enormous agenda-setting power and display the same bias in coverage as their counterparts in the mainstream political press.

Here's a random sampling of headlines from prominent, national publications:

"WHY VITAMIN PILLS DON'T WORK AND MAY BE BAD FOR YOU"

"STUDY: VITAMIN SUPPLEMENTS DON'T PROVIDE HEALTH BENEFITS"

"DO VITAMINS AND SUPPLEMENTS WORK? DOCTORS SAY NO"

**"MOST DIETARY SUPPLEMENTS DON'T DO ANYTHING.
WHY DO WE SPEND $35 BILLION A YEAR ON THEM?"**

Sound familiar?

To these we can add the phrase "expensive urine," commonly used in reference to supplements and as a way to dismiss any possibility of their value. We're not sure where that one originated but the implication is clear.

Consumers interested in improved health are left to wonder: Are vitamins good or bad? Should I take supplements?

The most accurate and truthful answer to these questions is one that most Americans don't want to hear: It depends.

As with most contentious debates, the topic of supplement use isn't black and white. The truth lies somewhere in the middle. The reality, though, is that Americans demand quick, simple answers. We move through life at such a frenetic pace, we rarely go beyond the headline. We may scan the bullet points but it's too much effort to drill down. We can't be bothered to perform any additional research, and we have no time to evaluate sources. We're too busy.

Unfortunately, with dietary supplements, there is no one-size-fits-all approach. There's no blanket response that will satisfy all parties. A 65-character headline cannot possibly capture the depth and breadth of some of these topics. To complicate things further—because there's profit potential involved—this particular subject lends itself to misinformation. The consumer suffers as a result. We become overwhelmed by the mixed messages.

The problem stems, in part, from word choice. The media often use the terms *vitamin* and *supplement* interchangeably. Perhaps this is done to simplify, but it is misleading and creates additional confusion. Here's the reality: All vitamins are supplements, but all supplements are not necessarily vitamins.

Let's establish some basic terminology. What are vitamins? Most of us are familiar with the letter vitamins: A, B, C, D, E, and maybe even K? There's a lot of buzz about magnesium these days, but that's not a vitamin, it's a mineral. And then there's curcumin. That's neither a vitamin nor a mineral, it's extracted from turmeric root. And what about antioxidants? Things like green tea extract and resveratrol? Is your head spinning yet?

Each of these has unique properties and varying degrees of evidence—from scant to comprehensive—that should be considered when assessing potential benefits and risks. Unfortunately, these compounds are often lumped together into the same category—vitamins—and our instinct is to paint all of them with that broad brush.

To be clear, this section of the book is not intended to provide specific recommendations or to advocate for or against *your* use of dietary supplements. Those decisions should be made in consultation with a qualified, nutritional-informed healthcare provider, and should be based on your health status.

My goal here is twofold:

1. **To highlight the limitations of vitamin studies.**

2. **To empower you, the reader, to be a more educated, discerning consumer.**

Lesson #1 should be clear already: look beyond the headline and beneath the surface!

You've got lots of options when shopping for supplements. Various brands, potencies, and delivery methods. Those differences matter. They determine the fate of the supplement you're digesting.

Form and dose are two of the most consequential factors dictating whether or not the supplement you swallow, spray, or apply to your skin gets where it needs to go to do what you want it to do.

Magnesium, for example, is available in at least a dozen forms. Now, if you're taking it for memory and brain health, you'd want a preparation known to cross the blood-brain barrier. Perhaps magnesium L-threonate. Those interested in heart health might go with magnesium orotate, which has been shown to improve cardiovascular function. Magnesium oxide, on the other hand, is the most poorly absorbed form of this mineral but it's cheap so it's often included in many multivitamin formulas.

Scientists refer to the absorption and use of a nutrient by the body as bioavailability. It's widely accepted that magnesium oxide has poor bioavailability so you would expect that a research study using that particular form of the mineral would lead to a different result than one that looks at magnesium citrate, which is known to be absorbed optimally. The magnesium oxide study would almost seem as if it were designed to fail.

Vitamin E presents a similar example. Vitamin E was long-touted for its health benefits, particularly in the prevention of cardiovascular disease. Then research emerged showing that vitamin E might increase the risk of lung cancer. The media promptly declared vitamin E supplementation to be dangerous, without acknowledging several flaws in the design of the study.

For starters, the study group was cigarette smokers, not exactly the healthiest population. The participants were using not just vitamin E but also supplemental beta carotene, a precursor to vitamin A. The form of vitamin E used in the study was the synthetic dl-alpha tocopheryl version, which is much less potent than the natural forms like d-alpha tocopherol or mixed tocopherols.

Clearly, even to a layperson, there were several confounding variables here that could explain the researchers' findings: Was it the vitamin E or the beta carotene that led to the increased cancer risk? Cigarettes contain carcinogens known to alter the DNA of cells in lung tissue—how much of a role did that play? Smokers tend to be less healthy in general. Were pre-existing conditions considered? And what about that synthetic form of vitamin E that was used? You'd be hard-pressed to find any recognition of these obvious study design flaws in the reporting on the vitamin E studies.

As it turns out, dozens of other studies demonstrate a beneficial effect from vitamin E supplementation, including a *reduced* risk of cancer. What do those studies have in common? They used the natural form of vitamin E.

Here's what one study determined to be the average risk reduction from a variety of causes of death among male smokers with the highest levels of *natural* vitamin E over a nearly 20-year period:

Disease	Mortality Reduction
Prostate cancer	32%
Ischemic stroke	37%
Hemorrhagic stroke	35%
Lung cancer	21%
Respiratory illness	42%

Many integrative cardiologists recommend natural vitamin E (or mixed tocopherols) to their heart patients due to its proven ability to prevent LDL cholesterol from becoming oxidized and unstable.

Vitamin D also appears in various forms. There's D2 (ergocalciferol) and D3 (cholecalciferol). D2 is what's most often used to fortify milk products but it's poorly absorbed and the body can't do much with it. D3 is the form of the vitamin that our bodies produce naturally when exposed to sunlight and is much better able to help us maintain beneficial levels of the vitamin in our bodies. Thus, D3 is the preferred version and the one that has been associated with a host of positive effects in hundreds of studies over many, many years.

Let's turn to supplementation with omega-3 fatty acids, or fish oil, one of the most well-researched nutraceuticals in history. There are three types of omega-3: eicosapentaenoic acid (EPA), docosahexaenoic acid (DHA), and alpha linolenic acid (ALA). EPA and DHA are found in fatty fish and available as supplements. ALA is a plant-based source of omega-3s prevalent in flaxseeds and walnuts and it's what a vegan would rely on for these fatty acids. The problem is that ALA has to first be converted to EPA and DHA before the body can use it. That conversion process is incredibly inefficient and results in very little of the most beneficial fatty acids being available. Hundreds of studies have shown a health benefit associated with an increased intake of omega-3 fatty acids, but mostly in the form of DHA and EPA.

While our governing agencies seem to be OK with fish oil supplementation (they even approved a pharmaceutical version), their recommended dose is a measly 500mg, far below the three to five grams shown to lead to improved mood and cardiovascular health. It's certainly valid to question if the higher dose is safe and that issue has been investigated. Toxicity studies—available to the media and known to researchers—have repeatedly demonstrated the absence of adverse effects using much, much higher doses. You would think this information would be of importance to any journalist writing on the topic.

Further, fish oil supplements are available primarily in two forms, based on the extraction and processing methods: triglyceride and ethyl ester. The former is much more easily absorbed and considered superior.

Studies are designed to investigate a specific hypothesis. Research has looked at the effect of fish oil supplementation on various risk factors for heart disease, of which there are nearly two dozen. Fish oil has been proven to address at least six of those risk factors, including elevated triglycerides and arrhythmia. However, when a study is designed to look at one of the other 16 risk factors, you might not expect fish oil to exert a beneficial effect. They waste no time in declaring:

"FISH OIL SUPPLEMENTS SHOWN TO BE USELESS; FAIL TO MEET PRIMARY ENDPOINT."

Well, of course they didn't meet the primary endpoint being examined in that study, but does that make them useless, which would be in complete contradiction to the conclusions of literally hundreds of other studies? Sleazy reporting? You decide.

Dose is another important consideration when evaluating the reliability of a vitamin study. Higher doses of fish oil, for example, confer impressive benefits in cardiovascular and brain health. Studies that use lower doses don't show much of an effect, yet somehow that's the research that the media chooses to highlight.

WHY THE ANTI-SUPPLEMENT BIAS?

It may surprise you to learn that doctors in the U.S. receive little to no training in nutrition while in medical school. A recent review reported that 71% of schools offer an average of only 19 hours of coursework in nutrition science over the course of a four-year program. Another finding was that fewer than 20% of schools offered even one class in nutrition.

Other analyses have shown that medical-school students are influenced by elements of the pharmaceutical industry from the time they arrive on campus. This appears in the form of aggressive advertising, as one example, and students in the past have even received gifts from these drug companies.

In one survey, a majority of medical school students said they remembered having been exposed to drug-company advertising 20 or more times. Another survey even showed that representatives from these companies were even being allowed to teach students in certain departments.

Upon graduating, these newly-minted physicians enter their profession having had no significance assigned to the role of diet and nutrition in disease, and having been ingrained with a pharmaceutical mindset, which gets reinforced each time they attend a medical conference.

Understandably, these overworked docs simply don't have the time to pursue advanced education in nutrition, nor do they recognize the need. That way of thinking is reflected in the quotes they provide when contacted by journalists asking them to weigh in on timely medical issues, such as the release of a new vitamin study.

It's hard for most conventionally trained doctors to think of natural remedies as being effective. We do emergency medicine really, really well in this country. Better than anyone. But we fail miserably when it comes to prevention—and that's where supplements come in.

Below is a look at some of the most persistent claims about supplement use and how they mislead unsuspecting consumers.

JUNK SCIENCE

* The anti-supplement crowd continues to argue that we can get all the nutrients we need from food.

REAL SCIENCE

* The typical Western diet today is characterized by excess sugar and fat, refined grain, processed meat, a lack of fiber, and a reliance on packaged foods. These empty calories provide little in the way of nutrition. Of the 3,600 calories the average American consumes each day, more than half of that is in the form of processed food.

According to recent data from the National Health and Nutrition Examination Survey (NHANES), the overwhelming majority of Americans don't eat the recommended amount of fruits and vegetables. The most commonly consumed? Lettuce (as an adornment on a hamburger), potatoes (in the form of the French fries that accompany that burger), and tomatoes (as in the tomato sauce that tops a slice of pizza).

It shouldn't surprise us, then, that the NHANES study came to the following conclusions about the nutrient status of the U.S. population, based on established daily requirements:

* 100% are deficient in potassium

* 94.3% are deficient in vitamin D

* 91.7% are deficient in choline

* 88.5% are deficient in vitamin E

* 66.9% are deficient in vitamin K

* 52.2% are deficient in magnesium

* 44.1% are deficient in calcium

* 43% are deficient in vitamin A

* 38.9% are deficient in vitamin C

While naysayers point to the fact that our ancestors didn't take supplements to justify their stance, this argument is also quite weak. Previous generations ate a varied, well-balanced diet. They didn't subsist on the convenience foods that define the standard American diet (SAD). Their vitamin D came from sun exposure and their "probiotics" from dirt.

The sad reality is that today's food supply bears little resemblance to that which nourished all manner of organisms through most of history. Our soil is dead, saturated with pH-altering, microbe-destroying chemical fertilizers, pesticides, and herbicides but depleted of minerals and other nutrients.

Most commercially available meat and dairy products come from animals raised on factory farms. The confinement on these feedlots invites bacterial infection and other illness, which is typically met with a regiment of antibiotics and other drugs. Those residues make their way through the food chain, potentially transmitting to our own microbiome. The resistant bugs can then damage the lining of the GI tract, contributing to the malabsorption of vitamins and minerals.

Some nutrient deficiencies stem from absorption issues related to celiac disease or many of the other gastrointestinal disorders that are increasingly common. Many Americans these days have chosen restricted ways of eating, in which entire food groups are eliminated. These include the paleolithic diets, ketogenic diets, carnivore, and vegan diets. As much as mainstream nutrition experts may advise against this, the phenomenon is real. The reality is that, even if we can get what we need from food, that's not what's happening.

JUNK SCIENCE

* Nutrient intake above the government's Recommended Daily Allowance (RDA) is unnecessary and possibly dangerous.

REAL SCIENCE

* The RDA is woefully inadequate, a situation that sensible supplementation can address.

These guidelines represent the minimum dose needed to stave off disease—scurvy in the case of vitamin C, and rickets for vitamin D, as two examples.

If you're reading this book, I'd venture to guess that you're interested in *optimal* wellness, that you're not content to merely hobble through life. That's the "why" in the title of this chapter.

The amount of a nutrient needed for longevity and enhanced quality of life is often vastly different from that which is needed simply to keep us alive. While the government tells us that 400 International Units (IU) of vitamin D per day is sufficient, the Vitamin D Council advises a daily intake of 4,000 IU, noting the absence of adverse effects up to 10,000 IU. Other groups make varying recommendations but the bulk of the evidence demonstrates that higher doses confer increased benefits:

* Rickets, reduced by 100%

* Osteomalacia, reduced by 100%

* Cancers, all combined, reduced by 75%

* Breast cancer, reduced by 50%

* Ovarian cancer, reduced by 25%

* Colon cancer, reduced by 67%

* Non-Hodgkins, reduced by 30%

* Kidney cancer, reduced by 67%

* Endometrial cancer, reduced by 35%

* Type 1 diabetes, reduced by 80%

* Type 2 diabetes, reduced by 50%

* Fractures, all combined, reduced by 50%

* Falls, women reduced by 72%

* Multiple Sclerosis, reduced by 50%

* Heart attack, men, reduced by 50%

* Peripheral vascular disease, reduced by 80%

* Preeclampsia reduced by 50%

* Cesarean section, reduced by 75

While sunlight may be the human body's preferred source of vitamin D, this method is only reliable in the absence of sunscreen, and the UV exposure involved may increase the risk of skin cancer. Further, for those living in northern climates, sunlight is too weak during parts of the year to allow for adequate vitamin D production. In this example, supplementation would be sensible.

The RDA is generic and provides no guidance for situations in which a certain population would require a higher nutrient intake. Vegetarians, for example, tend to be deficient in iron, iodine, and vitamin B12 and would therefore benefit from a supplement. Athletes have greater nutrient needs for recovery from physical activity in comparison to someone who leads a sedentary lifestyle. And someone battling cancer would have increased nutrient needs to help rebuild tissue and to maintain (or regain) weight.

JUNK SCIENCE

* Vitamins and supplements are not approved by the Food and Drug Administration (FDA) and therefore dangerous.

REAL SCIENCE

* This claim is misleading. Since 1994, the Food and Drug Administration has monitored the safety of dietary supplements, and continues to issue warnings to manufacturers, wholesalers, and distributors when illicit activity is discovered, and removes products from the market when they are suspected of being harmful. Further, FDA regulations prohibit supplement companies from making claims promising to prevent, treat, or cure any disease and requires this disclaimer be displayed on packaging. While supplements have a different classification in the eyes of government regulators, it's simply untrue to suggest that there's no oversight.

The truth is that prescription drugs are far more deadly than dietary supplements and those *are* FDA-approved. In its most recent report, the American Association of Poison Control Centers noted that not a single death had occurred in the U.S. in 2019 from the use of dietary supplements. Their review looked not only at vitamins and minerals, but also included herbal remedies and homeopathic formulas.

Further, of the emergency room visits attributed to supplement use, the majority were associated either with older adults having difficulty swallowing pills or with weight loss supplements. The latter represents a category known to commonly include *proprietary* blends. These often consist of stimulants and in undisclosed amounts. Unfortunately, those in the health press and academia who harbor anti-supplement biases will point to these rare instances as evidence of the danger of supplements as a whole.

The vast majority of deaths reported by the Poison Control Centers were from prescription and over-the-counter medications like acetaminophen. While pharmaceutical drugs are tested for safety, those studies are often short-term. A Phase 3 clinical trial, for example, lasts an average of three years. Compare that to the lengthy history of ascorbic acid (vitamin C), which has been produced since 1933.

The "FDA-approved" argument is also problematic given the agency's well-documented history of corruption. An investigation conducted by *Science* magazine found that a majority of agency regulators received financial support—including direct payments—from companies whose drugs they were to vote on.

This is the same agency that for years allowed the use of antibiotics in healthy animals as a means of growth promotion and the same agency that allows the use of food dyes such as FDC yellow 5 and 6 and other artificial colors that most of the rest of the world has seen fit to ban. In a 2006 survey of FDA scientists, 20% of respondents acknowledged being asked to omit information or alter documents. After the drug Vioxx was found to have caused up to 140,000 cases of heart disease (about half of those patients died), an FDA scientist testified to Congress that he was pressured to withhold safety information about the drug from the public.

START WITH DIET

- Even with all the nutrient depletion that has occurred over the past 50 years, there is still tremendous value in eating fruits and vegetables. You can maximize the nutrient density of your diet by choosing a wide-ranging, colorful variety of fruits and vegetables, preferably local and organically grown.

- Animal products should be pastured, grass-fed, and free-range to avoid exposure to toxins. Excess sugar, preservatives, and artificial flavors and dyes should be limited to avoid inflaming the gut and contributing to malabsorption. Traditional cooking fats should replace refined oils, as new evidence has shown that the omega-6 fatty acids like those found in corn and soybean oil can unfavorably alter our microbiome.

KNOW YOUR NUMBERS

- Work with a qualified, nutritionally-informed integrative or functional health practitioner to identify nutrient deficiencies, as well as genetic mutations such as methylenetetrahydrofolate reductase (MTHFR) that may impact nutrient metabolism. Testing for omega-3 status, and levels of B12, iron, and magnesium are particularly helpful. SpectraCell Laboratories offers one of the most comprehensive micronutrient panels. Supplement decisions should start with confirmed deficiencies.

- When shopping for supplements, stick with reputable brands. Some of the most respected include nutraMetrix, Thorne, Pure Encapsulations, Designs for Health, Klaire, Ortho Molecular, and Metagenics, all of which have been accredited by the Better Business Bureau. These and other professional labels are often used by university labs and other research institutions when conducting studies on nutrients.

- In general, companies that have survived in this competitive industry for at least 10 years are deemed more trustworthy than the many fly-by-night operations that seem to pop up weekly on Amazon.

- Buyer beware: while making purchases on Amazon may be convenient, a 2019 analysis by CNBC revealed that the company was selling expired products through third-party vendors. Amazon has also faced controversy in the past for the many counterfeit listings that have appeared on its platform over the last few years. For this reason, you may prefer to order directly from the manufacturer or through one of their verified consultants.

- You tend to get what you pay for. If a supplement seems too cheap, especially in comparison to other similar products, be suspicious.

- Use common sense, just as you would (or should) for any other type of purchase. Be cautious of any company that makes far-fetched, grandiose claims or offers free or discounted products in exchange for a positive review.

- Speaking of reviews: if they sound phony, they probably are, especially if there are thousands of them repeating the same type of praise. Websites like FakeSpot and ReviewMeta can help you analyze reviews for credibility.

- Patented forms of nutrients have usually been studied more extensively than their generic counterparts. Some examples include:

Kaneka® (CoQ10)

Carnipure® (L-carnitine tartrate)

ChromeMate® (chromium polynicotinate)

Kre-Alkalyn® (creatine)

BCM95®, Meriva®, C3® (curcumin)

MenaQ7® (K2 as MK7)

Sensori® or KSM-66® (ashwagandha)

Tonalin® (conjugated linoleic acid/CLA)

* Look for independent, third-party analyses that test for heavy metals and other contaminants. These include the following certifications: Good Manufacturing Practice (GMP), United States Pharmacopeia (USP), NSF, and International Fish Oil Standards (IFOS).

* Weigh *all* the evidence—or at least that which you can find and reasonably understand. If you've got a background in science or medicine and understand the difference between absolute and relative risk, you may enjoy spending some time on PubMed. For the rest of, some helpful online resources include Consumer Lab, Natural Medicines Comprehensive Database, and the Linus Pauling Micronutrient Research Center.

* Take the time to read the entire article, paying particular attention to what type of research was conducted, what the researchers were trying to find out, and how the study was designed. Actively seek out any criticism of the study or of the conclusion that was reached. Weigh the two and use common sense to decide who makes the stronger argument.

MIND THE DETAILS

* It's not always what you take but, rather, what you *absorb*. Be mindful of the form and dose of the nutrient, as well as the recommended frequency and how the supplement should be taken to allow for maximum absorption and assimilation.

* Fat-soluble nutrients must be taken with a fat-containing meal or snack. These include vitamins A, D, E, and K, as well as omega-3 and CoQ10 supplements. In contrast, water-soluble nutrients like vitamins B and C should be taken in a fasted state, about 30-60 minutes before or two to three hours after eating.

- Isotonic formulations are one of the best options available in terms of both absorption and potency. These are delivered in a state that allows them to be taken up directly by the small intestine for quick absorption into the bloodstream. With isotonics, your body absorbs roughly 95% of a nutrient, giving you much more bang for your buck. In comparison, the absorption rate for a supplement in pill or capsule form can be as low as 20%.

This chapter is not intended to be an indictment of the journalism profession, which has an important role to play here. Criticism is fine—helpful, in fact—as long as it's applied fairly and appropriately and not based on cherry-picked data.

The reality is that prescription drugs have their place. They can be effective and are sometimes necessary, but an honest review of the data informs us that supplements can sometimes reduce our reliance on medication, eliminate the need for them entirely or make them work better.

Critics of supplement use do make some valid claims. For example, there is growing evidence that some antioxidant supplements, when consumed in excess, can have unintended consequences, essentially acting as pro-oxidants in the body, increasing disease risk.

There's also concern that certain supplements can contribute to a cytokine "storm," a dangerous condition marked by an overproduction of immune cells.

And it's also true that many nutrients work better with a "supporting cast," as they are found in food and that this synergism is often lacking when nutrients are isolated in a lab for commercial sale.

An informed consumer is wise to look for misinformation coming at them from all directions. The inherent anti-supplement bias is dangerous but at the other end of the spectrum are the cure-alls, hocus pocus elixirs and potions being pushed by conspiracy theorists, self-appointed gurus, and other charlatans in every corner of the globe. These frauds make the credible practitioners in the natural health industry look bad, as some in the media and academia are unable-or unwilling- to distinguish between the two groups.

As I write this, one such group is promoting its Master Mineral Solution (MMS) as a cure for the current coronavirus pandemic. This concoction contains a bleaching agent, which is obviously dangerous. Kudos to the media for making us aware of this scam, but we've seen more than one press report that uses the very same article—the next paragraph, in fact—to criticize those who advocate the use of vitamin C, a proven antiviral and immune-booster and one that is currently being used with success in China with COVID patients.

In a perfect world, we'd get everything we need from food. The reality is that a truly balanced diet is rare and many Americans are suffering. Most of us take some type of nutraceutical. It's an industry worth several billions of dollars and that trend shows no sign of abating.

There's evidence that the medical school curriculum is changing to include more of an emphasis on healthy eating and the use of dietary supplements. A younger generation of American patients is demanding a shift from the band-aid approach of treating symptoms to a focus on holistic wellness and addressing root causes.

More promising still is the field of personalized nutrition, which is transforming how we go about achieving optimal wellness. Products such as the nutraMetrix Isotonix Custom Cocktail are customized to address an individual's specific needs. Customers are asked to complete a brief online questionnaire that covers health issues, diet, exercise, and current supplementation. The company then analyzes those responses to create an individualized supplement plan.

A new crop of doctors seems to get it. They are seeking advanced training in nutrition studies and they are more open-minded to the use of nutraceuticals to prevent and manage chronic illness. This gives us reason for optimism that we will once again have a partner in health. And record competition in the supplement industry has compelled manufacturers to increase transparency and adopt stricter standards. Regardless, disease prevention starts with the individual and ownership of the choices we make and how they impact our short- and long-term health.

Here's what we know, none of which is in dispute:

1. 60% of Americans have at least one chronic disease, which is the number one cause of death in the U.S and also the most costly.

2. Many chronic diseases can be prevented and managed with the appropriate dietary and lifestyle interventions.

3. Most Americans suffer from several nutrient deficiencies.

4. Many nutrient deficiencies can be corrected through supplementation.

Yes, there are some unscrupulous folks operating in the supplement business, but the same is true of the regulators that we trust to keep us safe. To unfairly malign an entire industry may be doing us more harm than good. Is denying informed consumers access to safe, proven supplements a form of malpractice? You decide.

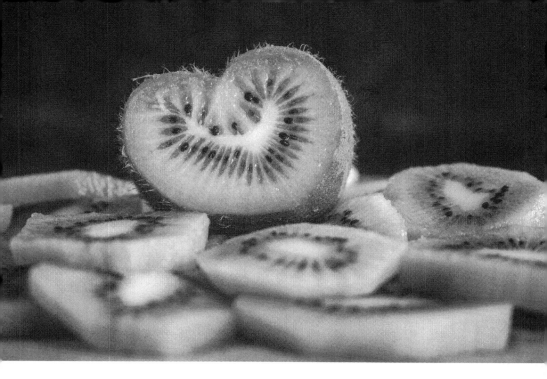

CHAPTER 09

Healthy Tummy, Healthy Heart

Data from the Centers for Disease Control and Prevention (CDC) show that someone in the United States has a heart attack every 40 seconds. And every 60 seconds, at least one person dies from a heart disease-related event.

Cardiovascular diseases are the leading cause of death in the world, with coronary heart disease—the most common type—accounting for 1 in 7 deaths in the United States. As more than half of us are walking around with at least one risk factor for the disease, it's no surprise that the World Health Organization has predicted it will remain the primary cause of death from chronic disease for years to come.

Then there's the economic toll. The CDC has determined that heart disease costs the United States more than $200 billion each year. This sum includes the cost of healthcare services, medications, and lost productivity.

Despite our decades-long education in "heart-healthy" living and modern advances in diagnosis and treatment, the heart disease mortality rate is on the rise, particularly among young people. In 2019, heart disease was responsible for 25% of American deaths.

What are we to make of this? Are we falling behind in the battle to prevent heart disease? Why? For years, this conversation has focused almost entirely on lipids and lipoproteins, despite the fact that most major heart attacks occur in people who have *normal* cholesterol.

The so-called lipid theory—the idea that an overindulgence in dietary cholesterol leads to atherosclerosis—has persisted for more than half a century. More and more studies, however, have exposed the flawed reasoning and imperfect science that formed the basis of that framework. This has forced a paradigm shift, with an increasing number of doctors questioning the assertion that effective management of arterial disease requires lowering cholesterol, especially with statins—a $30 billion per year industry.

Conventional medicine recognizes a set of *traditional* risk factors for heart disease that include not only dyslipidemia, but also age, hypertension, diabetes, obesity, smoking, and a lack of exercise.

While these predispositions should be a part of any cardiovascular risk assessment, there's clearly a missing piece to this puzzle. For example, what *causes* hypertension? Or diabetes? Or cholesterol issues? What if the solution to our health problems is already inside our bodies?

As you read this, there are trillions of bacteria swimming in your colon. Indeed, gut function has been one of the hottest topics in health research over the past two decades.

The Human Microbiome Project (HMP) was launched in 2007 by the National Institutes of Health to study the relationship between humans and the intestinal flora we host.The aim was to learn more about microbes and the differences between a healthy and diseased state in the gut.

The findings of the HMP suggest that it is more likely than ever that the microbiome is just as consequential to our health as our DNA, if not more so. While our genes are inherited and can't be changed, continuing advances allow us to alter the microbiome in ways that may improve our health.

A link between the gut and metabolism has been demonstrated. Same for immunity. The gut-brain connection has been established and we've seen evidence of a gut-skin interplay. It really shouldn't surprise us, then, that a gut-heart axis has emerged.

It has been observed that the guts of heart patients host more of the inflammatory microbes known to promote atherosclerosis. The microbiome of healthy individuals, on the other hand, have strains of bacteria such as Bacteroides and others that produce anti-inflammatory molecules, such as butyric acid.

Researchers have known for quite some time that oxidative stress and inflammation harm the arteries as we age, but the exact trigger has remained somewhat of a mystery. As it turns out, an aging gut produces toxic molecules that damage tissue.

But exactly *how* do these gut pathogens make us sick? There are at least four mechanisms through which gut health can impact your risk of heart disease.

GUT-HEART LINK #1:
SMALL INTESTINE BACTERIAL OVERGROWTH (SIBO)

SIBO is characterized by an overgrowth of normal—or *good*—bacteria in the small intestine, rather than in the colon where they should be located. Recent studies have suggested that SIBO could be the cause of most cases of irritable bowel syndrome (IBS), a condition that affects more than 20% of Americans.

Research has demonstrated a strong correlation between people found to have small intestinal bacterial overgrowth (SIBO) and coronary artery disease (CAD). In one study, 1,059 patients were screened for SIBO using breath test. Patients who tested positive had a significantly higher incidence of CAD as well as a higher incidence of diabetes and chronic kidney disease.

It is clear that patients with SIBO should be classified as high risk for a cardiac event and will want to aggressively control other risk factors, such as hypertension or diabetes.

THE ROLE OF NUTRIENT DEFICIENCIES

The symptoms of SIBO and IBS are largely the same and include diarrhea, constipation, gas, bloating, and nutrient deficiencies due to poor digestion or absorption. Such deficiencies likely explain, at least in part, the link to heart disease.

The overgrowth of bacteria in SIBO patients damages the intestinal lining, making the surface permeable and creating a situation commonly referred to as *leaky gut*. The bacteria consume nutrients such as water-soluble B vitamins like B6 (pyridoxine) and B12 before our own cells have a chance to. This creates a deficiency and is often seen in patients who suffer with GI problems.

Vitamins B6 and B12, along with folate, are known to lower the body's levels of homocysteine, a strong indicator of heart disease risk and associated death. Deficiency of these vitamins contributes to a variety of atherogenic processes, including arterial damage and clotting in the blood vessels.

Another B vitamin—pantethine—may help reduce the oxidation of LDL cholesterol and, in clinical trials, has led to significant improvements in triglycerides and HDL.

The bacteria may also decrease fat absorption through their effect on bile acids, leading to deficiencies in fat-soluble nutrients like vitamin D. Mounting research has identified low vitamin D status as a risk factor for cardiovascular disease, and related issues such as high blood pressure and diabetes.

Italian researchers recently reported that vitamin D may improve the lining of blood vessel walls to enhance blood flow and may counter the dangerous effects of inflammation. A 2017 study out of Ohio University showed that vitamin D could *reverse* some of the damage to the heart and blood vessels caused by high blood pressure.

Among fat-soluble nutrients, vitamin K—and K2, specifically—has been increasingly recognized as a cardiovascular protector. K2 activates Matrix Gla Protein (MGP), which prevents calcium from depositing in the blood vessels. SIBO is associated with reduced MGP activation and a resulting arterial stiffening.

The standard American diet is quite low in K2 so we must rely on our guts to produce what we need. Those with gut dysfunction have an impaired ability to synthesize K2, leaving them more at risk for atherosclerosis.

Coenzyme Q10 (CoQ10) behaves like a vitamin and is found in every cell in the body but is most heavily concentrated in the heart, where it assists in energy production. CoQ10 has been shown in studies to reduce blood pressure and has led to improvements in patients with cardiomyopathy. Research has demonstrated a strong relationship between severity of heart disease and low CoQ10 levels. Like vitamins D and K, CoQ10 is fat-soluble and SIBO patients may be deficient.

Nutrient depletion is only one pathway through which poor gut health contributes to the development of heart disease. Systemic, chronic inflammation is caused by bad bacteria leaking through intestinal lining. Inflammation damages the arteries.

In contrast to the acute inflammation by which the body fights infections and heals, this sustained, low level of inflammation irritates the blood vessels. This process sets the stage for a heart attack by increasing the buildup of plaque, which can then break open and form a clot.

Besides protecting the body against dangerous levels of homocysteine, vitamin B6 also tames inflammation in the gut. Low B6 levels correlate strongly with high levels of chronic inflammation. Conversely, people with the highest vitamin B6 levels in the blood have the lowest levels of inflammation.

SIBO is more prevalent than previously thought and because subclinical atherosclerosis can result, aggressive action may be needed to address the issue.

THE URBAN BODY FIX

* First, get a **diagnosis**. The symptoms of SIBO overlap with many other gut disorders and medical conditions. There are currently a number of diagnostic tests available to screen for SIBO.

    1. A breath test measures levels of hydrogen and methane, both byproducts of the fermentation associated with an overgrowth of bacteria in the small intestines. Unfortunately, the accuracy of breath tests has been questioned and false negative and false positive results occur fairly often.

    2. Endoscopies are sometimes performed to diagnose SIBO but these procedures are both invasive and costly.

3. A third method would involve a trial of antibiotics. Rifaximin is usually the first choice, as it stays in the gut and out of the bloodstream so side effects are much less of a concern.

- Many patients experience a recurrence of symptoms after treatment with antibiotics, making the pharmaceutical approach less than ideal. From a functional medicine perspective, the root cause must be identified before lasting relief can be expected.

- Assuming that anatomical abnormalities can be ruled out, SIBO patients should be assumed to have low stomach acid. This condition—along with age—can increase gastric pH levels, allowing for bacterial overgrowth.

- Avoid long-term use of the following:

  1. **Proton pump inhibitors (PPIs).** These may cause a B12 deficiency, as well as infection with Clostridium difficile (C. diff) bacterium. Patients on omeprazole have higher levels of "bad" bacteria like Enterococcus, Streptococcus, Staphylococcus, and some strains of E. coli.

  2. **Non-steroidal anti-inflammatory drugs (NSAIDs)** like ibuprofen can damage the intestinal lining, cause inflammation, and contribute to leaky gut.

  3. **Narcotic pain medications.** Opioids slow gut activity, leading to constipation, nausea, and vomiting, especially in those with underlying IBS.

- **Low bile flow** and **enzyme deficiencies** are also common causes of SIBO. Adequate bile promotes the growth of gut bacteria while keeping it where it should be and is important to prevent and reverse SIBO. Bile acids also seal up a leaky gut.

- Bile deficiency is usually a result of liver or gallbladder dysfunction but its proper flow can be supported with supplemental **phosphatidylcholine** (PS). In addition, PS may help protect the mucus layer of the digestive tract, lower inflammation, and repair some of the damage caused by the overuse of NSAIDs.

* Nutrient deficiencies common among SIBO patients should be addressed through diet first.

    Vitamin A: Cod liver oil, eggs, squash, sweet potato, carrots, spinach, broccoli, and red pepper

    Vitamin B12: fish, meat, poultry, eggs, and milk product

    Vitamin E: nuts and seeds

    Vitamin K2: meat, eggs, and dairy, preferably from grass-fed or pastured animals

    Omega-3 fatty acids: fatty fish, such as salmon, sardines, and mackerel

* The use of dietary supplements is sometimes more appropriate to ensure a beneficial dose of each nutrient and in a form the body can optimally assimilate. These include vitamin D and co-enzyme Q10 (CoQ10). Supplemental vitamin E—in its high-gamma form or as mixed tocopherols—has antioxidant properties, protecting cholesterol particles from oxidation and increasing the number of LDL receptors to help with its removal by the liver.

* One note of caution when it comes to supplements: patients who have a history of SIBO are advised to limit probiotic use to yeast-based strains like **Saccharomyces boulardii** (commonly marketed as Florastor) that cannot overgrow in the small bowel.

* Research has shown that restricting fermentable oligo-, di-, and monosaccharides, and polyols (FODMAPs) can ease the symptoms associated with SIBO and related GI disorders. High-FODMAP foods include many that are hard to avoid, particularly when dining out: wheat, garlic, onions, and popular fruits and vegetables, such as broccoli, mushrooms, peas, apples, and peaches.

* Serving size and degree of ripeness are factors, with smaller portions and less ripeness sometimes turning a high-FODMAP food into a low- or moderate-FODMAP food. A **low-FODMAP** diet is obviously quite restrictive and should serve only as a template. It's recommended that patients work with a registered dietitian (RD) to identify specific intolerances and to customize a diet based on their needs.

* Foods should always be reintroduced one at a time and gradually, taking note of any adverse reactions to identify sensitivities.

GUT-HEART LINK #2: HELICOBACTER PYLORI (H. PYLORI)

H. pylori is a very common bacterial infection and the cause of most stomach ulcers. It is very contagious and can be spread through food, water, and fecal contamination. H. pylori can also be transmitted in the saliva or bodily fluids of those who are infected. It's more prevalent in parts of the world known for poor sanitation.

Most people with H. pylori have no symptoms. If the infection progresses to an ulcer, patients may experience abdominal pain, diarrhea, decreased appetite, and fatigue.

H. pylori has only recently been identified as a risk factor for heart disease after being found within plaque in the arteries of heart patients. In a 2005 study published in Heart, Italian researchers discussed their finding that people with atrial fibrillation were 20 times more likely to test positive for H. pylori, than people without the condition.

Infection with H. pylori also appears to:

* Accelerate and worsen atherosclerosis

* Increase the risk of heart attack and stroke

* Increase the risk and severity of angina

* Cause or worsen dyslipidemia

* Increase insulin resistance

* Increase blood pressure

- Increase C-Reactive Protein (CRP), a measure of systemic inflammation

- Increase oxidative stress

- Increase homocysteine

- Increase fibrinogen

- Result in nutritional deficiencies

The obvious question is how? Although still controversial, several potential mechanisms have been proposed:

1. In adults, H. pylori triggers an active chronic inflammatory process, perhaps weakening the stability of plaque in the arteries.

2. Infection by H. pylori induces an elevation of triglyceride levels with a decrease in HDL cholesterol, both being cardiovascular risk factors.

3. Some researchers suggest that the production of oxidants—compounds that damage cellular DNA—is also important. It has been observed that antioxidant levels decrease in patients with H. pylori, possibly causing blood vessel and tissue damage and setting the stage for atherogenesis.

(Contrary to conventional medical thinking, we now know that it is oxidized low density lipoproteins (LDL) cholesterol specifically that is one of the primary causes of atherosclerosis and not the condition of having too much cholesterol in general.)

H. pylori can be detected with blood, breath, and stool tests.

H. pylori infections usually require a combination treatment consisting of two antibiotics and a proton pump inhibitor (PPI). These medications can cause side effects and this regimen has been less effective of late due to drug resistance.

Fortunately, there are natural therapies that can be helpful in preventing these side effects, protecting the stomach, helping the body to better fight infection, and promoting overall good health. However, these natural treatments won't completely rid your body of H. pylori, so you may decide to use them as a complementary strategy.

* In one study, **honey**—particularly the Manuka variety—was shown to inhibit the growth of H. pylori in gastric cells.

* Research conducted on both animal and human subjects has demonstrated the beneficial effects of sulforaphane against H. pylori bacteria. This powerful detoxifying compound is responsible for the health-promoting benefits of cruciferous vegetables. **Broccoli sprouts** are one of the best sources of vsulforaphane in the diet.

* Studies have shown that the **probiotics** Lactobacillus, Bifidobacterium, and Saccharomyces boulardii fight H. pylori by competing with the bacteria to adhere to the mucosal lining of the stomach.

* A study published in 2009 in the *Journal of Nutrition* reported that supplementing with the amino acid **l-glutamine** may enhance the immune response to H. pylori infection in its initial stages.

* Research has shown that the combination of **oregano oil** and **cranberry extract** work synergistically to inhibit H. pylori.

Some animal products—red meat, egg yolks, dairy, and fish—contain the nutrients choline and l-carnitine, which the gut breaks down into a compound called trimethylamine (TMA). The liver then converts TMA to trimethylene N-oxide, or TMAO.

Higher TMAO levels put you at greater risk for heart disease. In fact, TMAO has been linked to a 62% increased likelihood of plaque formation and atherosclerosis.

Red meat and fish appear to raise TMAO levels much more than poultry and eggs. Fish consumption has long been associated with longevity so it's likely that the beneficial compounds in fish counteract some of the harmful effects of TMAO.

The exact mechanism is still being investigated but researchers think TMAO influences cholesterol and bile acid metabolism, triggers inflammation, stimulates the creation of foam cells in the walls of blood vessels, and increases the risk of clot formation. The more our gut is exposed to red meat, the more TMA-producing bacteria it develops. Interestingly, it's been observed that vegans and vegetarians have very few of these microbes and are thus unable to produce much TMA in the gut or TMAO in the liver—at least initially.

There is a blood test available for TMAO but this isn't yet included in a standard cardiovascular risk panel. That may change as research in this area evolves.

THE URBAN BODY FIX

* Don't panic! TMAO is just one of many, many risk factors for heart disease. That being said, if you're a heavy meat-eater, you now have another reason to cut back and to consider a more **plant-based diet**.

- One study demonstrated that **resveratrol**—an antioxidant found in the skin of red grapes—can alter the bacteria in the gut in such a way that TMA formation is inhibited and TMAO levels reduced.

- A compound (dimethyl butanol) in **extra virgin olive oil** and **red wine vinegar** may block the enzyme that produces TMAO.

- **Cruciferous vegetables** (broccoli, kale, cabbage, cauliflower) suppress the activity of the FMO3 enzyme that plays a key role in converting TMA to TMAO.

GUT-HEART LINK #4: LEPTIN RESISTANCE

Leptin is a hormone produced by fat tissue and specialized cells in the small intestines. Its primary role is to inhibit hunger and reduce fat storage but it also has major effects on gastrointestinal function and leptin receptors have been identified in the cardiovascular system and in coronary arteries.

Studies have shown that higher circulating leptin levels are associated with a greater risk of coronary heart failure and cardiovascular disease. Clinical and population studies have found a correlation between high levels of circulating leptin and the abnormal enlargement, or thickening, of the heart muscle, particularly in obese patients.

We also know that leptin impacts the remodeling of the heart and the blood vessels, which can contribute to arrhythmias, as well as the development and progression of heart failure.

Leptin plays a key role in the circulation of blood, oxygen, and nutrients from the heart to organs and tissues. Some of those actions are thought to promote the formation of fatty plaques in the arteries, and possibly the formation of a clot within the blood vessels.

Leptin may trigger inflammation, oxidative stress, and a thickening of the blood vessels. These changes can restrict blood flow and contribute to the development or progression of diabetes, hypertension, atherosclerosis, and coronary heart disease.

ADOLSTERONE

It also appears that leptin triggers the production of the steroid hormone aldosterone. High aldosterone levels contribute to systemic inflammation, blood vessel stiffness, enlarged heart, and insulin resistance.

Aldosterone, which is made in the adrenal gland, directly impacts blood pressure by regulating salt-water balance in the body. High levels of aldosterone are very common in obesity patients and a primary cause of cardiovascular issues.

LEPTIN RESISTANCE

Under normal circumstances, leptin induces a feeling of fullness, letting us know that it's time to stop eating. When certain receptors in the brain no longer respond to that signal, we're thought to be suffering from leptin resistance. Higher leptin levels are associated with increased fat mass. This may explain the link between heart disease and obesity.

THE URBAN BODY FIX

* The relationship between a fish diet or a vegetarian diet and leptin was studied in an African population. In both men and women, **fish consumption** is associated with lower plasma leptin levels than are vegetable diets.

* The probiotic **Lactobacillus** reduces leptin and improves heart function.

* You can increase leptin sensitivity by **avoiding inflammatory foods** like sugar and trans fat.

* **Regular resistance training** and **aerobic exercise** both reduce leptin levels, increase leptin sensitivity, and lead to improvements in lipid metabolism.

Despite considerable progress, our understanding of the microbiome in health and human disease is still a relatively young science. Certainly, we can expect some exciting breakthroughs in the coming years. What can we do right now? Quite a bit, as it turns out.

That starts with staying on top of GI issues, including gas and bloating. If they persist, that could be a warning sign and getting the right diagnosis is crucial.

Though antibiotics are commonly used—and sometimes necessary—to address dysbiosis, these drugs can do more harm than good. Treatment through dietary manipulation and lifestyle change, however, comes without side effects.

Results from genetic studies reveal that hereditary factors account for only 15% of heart disease risk. The remainder is environmental and the biggest part of that is diet, which is modifiable. While drugs act in a more systemic way, dietary modification allows use to be more targeted.

* It is common, for example, for patients with SIBO to have food intolerances, especially to carbohydrates. Aside from experimenting with carbohydrate restriction, consider **testing for food intolerances**. I recommend the Multiple Food Immune Reactivity Screen (Array 10) from Cyrex Labs.

* **Limit refined sugar** and **carbohydrates**, which decrease the amount of friendly bacteria in the gut, feed harmful bacteria, and increase body-wide inflammation.

* Some foods have been shown to help. **Walnuts**, for example, promote good bacteria (Eubacterium eligens, Lachnospiraceae).

* Although scientific evidence is lacking, some people find that drinking **apple cider vinegar** every day is an effective natural remedy for low stomach acid.

* **FACT**: Heart disease patients who **eat more fiber** experience less death and less need for transplants. Research has shown that fiber can help lower a person's risk of heart disease. **Psyllium** is a good option and can benefit your heart by reducing blood pressure, improving lipid levels, and strengthening the heart muscle.

- Short chain fatty acids (SCFAs) are particularly helpful and these come from fiber. SCFA are by-products of fermentation found in the intestinal tract and the primary energy source for the cells that line your colon. You can increase levels of SCFA by consuming more resistant starch in the form of cooked and cooled potatoes and rice, green bananas and plantains, white beans, and oats.

- Eat more fruits and vegetables. It might sound cliche but these non-digestible carbohydrates reach the colon almost entirely intact and promote bacterial diversity. It's known that heart failure patients have less diversity in their guts.

- Fermented foods like kimchi, sauerkraut, yogurt, and kefir provide probiotic strains that lower inflammatory markers (TNF-alpha, C-reactive protein) and increase the production of nitric oxide, which relaxes blood vessels and lowers blood pressure.

- **Inulin** is a prebiotic, which are naturally occurring compounds found in garlic, onions, asparagus, and Jerusalem artichokes, among other foods. **Prebiotics** work by promoting the growth of the beneficial bacteria in the large intestine, which inhibits the growth of pathogens such as *C. difficile* and *E. coli*. Inulin and other prebiotics are fermented in the colon and produce **short chain fatty acids** (SCFA). These increase the absorption of water, sodium, and electrolytes from the gut, which may ease GI symptoms such as diarrhea.

- **A high-salt diet changes gut composition.** Research published in the journal *Nature* found that too much sodium in the diet reduced levels of Lactobacillus bacteria in mice, which led to a greater number of immune cells associated with high blood pressure.

- Animal protein has been linked to infectious bacteria and a **plant-based diet** seems to be protective. Accordingly, gut diversity is highest among herbivores and lowest in carnivores.

- Vegetable oils (corn, sunflower, cottonseed, safflower) induce stomach inflammation. Instead, opt for traditional cooking fats or those with a favorable Omega-6:Omega-3 ratio: **olive oil**, **coconut oil**, **avocado oil**.

- **Exercise** increases the population and diversity of good bacteria in the gut.

> **All disease begins in the gut.**

It's been more than 2,000 years since Hippocrates famously made this claim, and it's becoming increasingly clear that—at least in the case of a *leaky* gut—he may have been right. While the importance of gut health has been largely ignored by mainstream medicine, research is finally catching up.

At least 70 million Americans struggle with some type of gastrointestinal disorder. For many of those people, the symptoms are merely a source of mild to moderate discomfort but the potential long-term implications are far more serious.

The science of gut health may be in its infancy, but truly cutting-edge, individualized, and holistic treatments are on the horizon. It's looking increasingly likely that, someday, a swab, stool sample, or breath test will be able to predict heart disease risk. In the meantime, we can take responsibility for our health, empowered with proactive strategies like those discussed above.

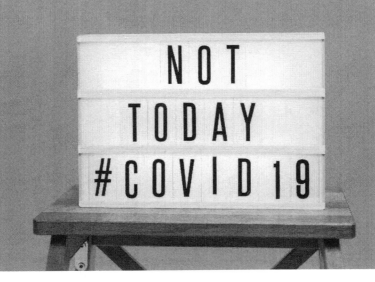

CHAPTER 10

Natural Immunity in the Pandemic Age

Even before the outbreak of COVID-19, Americans had become increasingly interested in natural immune boosters. That's a positive development. Unfortunately, this newly found focus on proactive wellness also leaves us prey to unscrupulous marketers and the many cure-alls they're peddling all over the Web. The good news is that there are many safe, proven preventative measures we can take to protect ourselves—in some cases, without spending a penny.

While frequent hand-washing and social distancing remain the most effective means of preventing the spread of coronavirus and other contagious diseases, we can also trust our innate immune system to recognize and defend against foreign invaders. This assumes that we do our part in arming it with the necessary tools. The other side of that equation is an avoidance of immune-suppressing activity.

Before we get to the nuts and bolts of immune system strengthening, a quick primer is in order.

—————— **IMMUNITY 101**

You probably don't need convincing that the immune system is an integral part of the human defense system. On guard 24/7 against all manner of foreign invaders, our immune system is tasked with our survival. It goes about this monumental task by means of a division of labor, which we will discuss now.

When we talk about immune function, we're actually referring to two different systems, each designed to contribute in its own way. The innate immune system kicks in immediately in response to a virus, bacteria, parasite, or other pathogen inside the body. Innate immunity relies on physical barriers—skin, hair, mucus, saliva—to prevent the spread of any foreign invaders. On the surface of these pathogens is a substance known as an antigen, which triggers a generalized response by the innate immune system. This could manifest itself in the form of inflammation or an allergic reaction, among other examples.

If the innate immune system is unable to control the spread of a pathogen, the adaptive immune system kicks in. Also referred to as acquired immunity, this system sometimes requires days or weeks after the initial innate reaction before mounting a specialized attack against a virus, bacteria, or other pathogen. Once the adaptive immune system responds, it then commits its enemy to *memory*, a feature that allows for long-term protection. If the same pathogen is recognized in the future, the adaptive immune system will launch an even stronger attack.

Readers of this book will no doubt be aware that most of our immune system resides in the gut. However, parts of the immune system are located elsewhere in the body. These areas are the lymphatic system, the thymus, the spleen, and the bone marrow. Each of these organs stores white blood cells, or leukocytes. That's where we'll turn our attention now.

There are two categories of white blood cells—phagocytes and lymphocytes—and each of those consists of several subtypes.

INNATE IMMUNE SYSTEM

PHAGOCYTES

1. **Neutrophils:**

    - Are the most common and abundant type of white blood cell

    - Are made in bone marrow and circulate in the bloodstream

    - Are the first cells to respond to a bacterial infection

    - Surround and digest foreign invaders (viruses, bacteria, parasites)

    - Have a very short lifespan

2. **Macrophages:**

    - Are also *first responders*

    - Can also engulf and eat a foreign invader

    - Present antigens to T cells

- Trigger an inflammatory response by releasing cytokines, which recruits other immune cells

- Can survive for months

3. **Natural killer (NK) cells:**

- Circulate and surveil for infected cells

- Can tell the difference between healthy and unhealthy cells

- Attach to an abnormal cell—especially cancer cells—and inject it with chemicals

- Can kill spontaneously and doesn't need to be activated first

4. **Dendritic cells:**

- Serve as a link between innate and adaptive immune system

- Carry antigens on their surface and present them to T cells, activating adaptive immune response

ADAPTIVE IMMUNE SYSTEM

LYMPHOCYTES

1. **B cells:**

- Produce antibodies, proteins that can attach to a specific invader and mark it to alert other cells

2. **T cells:**

- Learn to recognize and destroy abnormal cells

- Also release cytokines

- Recruit other immune cells

As you can see, the immune system is complex. Comparisons to an army or police force are apt. The above components—and many others—work together intricately to protect us. When it's operating as it should, you won't even notice. But what if there's a problem? Signs of immune dysfunction may or may not be obvious. These may include fatigue, digestive issues, frequent infections, or slow healing of wounds. Underlying most of this—and most chronic disease—is a state of ongoing, systemic inflammation.

Where does the inflammation come from? It's triggered when the immune system reacts to something in our body. If it's something we're allergic to, then cytokines are released, and genes are activated in specific immune cells. This can manifest itself in the form of rashes,eczema, or sinus issues, and those can be an indication that your immune system has been thrown off and that there might be some kind of imbalance.

Many factors influence immune function. Heredity plays a role, and while our DNA is unalterable, a genetic predisposition doesn't seal your medical fate. Genes don't act in isolation. Some genes can only do us harm once activated. Genes can also be *silenced*. As it turns out, there are many diet and lifestyle factors with access to that ON/OFF switch. And that's where we have nearly complete control. It's incumbent upon us to be good stewards of our bodies and the *Urban Body Fix* philosophy is firmly rooted in the concept of personal responsibility.

On that note, we'll now focus on these modifiable factors and the role they play in immune function and disease risk.

DIET—EAT LESS OF THESE:

◦ SUGAR

The U.S. government estimates that the average American eats over 150 *pounds* of sugar each year! This is easy to accomplish considering that 75% of the food on grocery store shelves contains added sugars. Many of these are disguised with unrecognizable names and hidden in unsuspected places (bread, ketchup, salad dressing). The damage this inflicts goes well beyond weight gain and dental cavities.

The link between sugar consumption and the immune system is complex and there's much we don't understand. What is clear, however, is that sugar is more than simply a form of energy that gets used up during physical activity. That idea is antiquated but, unfortunately, many still hold that view.

Here's what we know: Sugar from the diet feeds bad bacteria and inhibits immunity. It does this by making the neutrophils less aggressive in going after the bad guys, at least in the case of bacteria. There's evidence that sugar may behave differently in the presence of viral infection.

Excess sugar intake can also have an indirect impact on immune function. High-sugar foods have fewer nutrients and a deficiency in certain vitamins and minerals makes you more susceptible to illness.

Calories from sugar also make it easier to over-consume those foods, which can lead to weight gain. Research has established that overweight individuals tend to suffer from weakened immunity. We've also learned that both diabetic and overweight patients are more susceptible to COVID-19. Perhaps too much sugar in the blood is a risk factor.

So how much sugar is *too* much? One study out of Loma Linda University found that 75 grams inhibits the activity of white blood cells by as much as 50%. This is the amount found in two cans of soda. The same researchers observed that this immune dysfunction begins 30-60 minutes after consumption and lasts for up to five hours.

VEGETABLE OIL

This one flies under the radar, even among many nutrition experts. To be clear, we're talking about corn, safflower, sunflower, soybean, and cottonseed oil. We've been told for years that these unsaturated fats were better for heart health but more recent studies have demonstrated the opposite effect. The omega-6 fatty acids found in these oils can actually damage the arteries, increasing the risk of atherosclerosis. It is through the same mechanism that vegetable oil inhibits immunity. But how? Here comes that "I" word again: **inflammation**.

As discussed in other parts of this book, our fatty acid intake needs to be balanced in order for us to achieve optimal health. Through most of human history, that ratio was about 3:1, Omega-6:Omega-3. Today, that number is closer to 20:1, a testament to the rise of industrial food processing. A modern Western diet is characterized by its reliance on convenience foods. Most of our vegetable oil consumption today is in the form packaged foods like chips, crackers, and baked goods.

Our increased consumption of omega-6 fatty acids parallels the rise in the diagnoses of many chronic, degenerative diseases, from cancer and Alzheimer's to irritable bowel syndrome and autoimmunity. And much of that can be attributed to the skewed ratio of fatty acids that typifies the standard American diet. While some are required by the body, excess omega-6's activate genes that promote inflammation. This marks the initial step in an immune response that will often run amok.

Further, these industrial seed oils are highly processed, often with damaging heat and the use of solvents like hexane. *Deodarization* is actually one of the many steps involved in producing canola oil. This involves using chemicals to mask the smell of some of the powerful compounds used in the process of turning a rapeseed (there's no such thing as a canola plant) into something we're told we should be putting in our bodies. The increased use of genetically modified organisms (GMOs) further confuses our immune system.

By now you've realized that *Urban Body Fix* is predicated on a holistic approach.

Research has confirmed the effect of emotional and psychological stress on the immune system. In several studies, questionnaires were used to assess the stress levels of students prior to taking an exam. Measures of T cell response and interferon gamma (an activator of macrophages) were consistently shown to have decreased, resulting in "significant" immune suppression, according to these researchers.

It's also been established that stress can trigger flare-ups of digestive disorders.

While the term is most often associated with feelings of anxiety and fear, stress can also come in the form of the *physical* tension we inflict upon our bodies. In the right dose and at the appropriate intensity, exercise has many desirable effects on the immune system. The body interprets this short-term physiological stressor as a need to ramp up its defenses. The immune system sends out armies of neutrophils and lymphocytes to monitor for and eliminate any pathogens.

A 2010 study published in the *British Journal of Sports Medicine* found that adults who exercise for 20 minutes or more at least five days each week experienced 43% fewer days with upper respiratory infections than participants who abstained from exercise. Study participants who did report getting sick found their symptoms to be milder.

On the other end of the spectrum are the chronic exercisers, a group whose activity level, frequency, and intensity produces unintended consequences. Gym rats and exercise junkies may be familiar with the symptoms of overtraining syndrome: fatigue, frequent injuries, reduced motivation, mood issues, and a drop off in performance. More common among athletes, overtraining is associated with elevated levels of the stress hormone cortisol.

Produced by the adrenal glands, cortisol does some good in the body, regulating blood sugar, blood pressure, metabolism, and inflammation. Cortisol prepares us for physical activity by raising blood sugar levels and activating our *fight-or-flight* response. Shortly after the completion of a bout of exercise, cortisol levels should return to baseline. Lengthy and high-intensity activities (without proper recovery) can lead to chronically elevated cortisol levels and a corresponding suppression of immune function. The mechanism here is an increase in inflammatory cytokines. Maybe this explains why competitive runners are more prone to upper respiratory infections, especially in the days after a race.

● ALCOHOL

While many sectors of the economy have been dealt a major blow by the COVID-19 pandemic, sales of alcoholic beverages were up 55% a couple of months into the quarantine compared to the same period the previous year. Nielsen Research reported a 243% increase in online sales during a stretch of March 2020. And in surveys, roughly one-third of respondents working remotely admitted to drinking every day *while on the job!* Alcohol-on-demand home delivery services make it easier than ever to self-medicate.

Though no research has specifically looked at alcohol consumption and immune function as it relates to COVID-19, previous studies have shown that alcohol disrupts the balance of microbes in the gut, depleting us of the beneficial bacteria that would otherwise help fight off an infection. Alcohol is also known to irritate the immune cells that make up our airways, allowing pathogens easier access. Even when consumed within recommended guidelines, alcohol intake can depress immune function. Alcohol also indirectly lowers immunity by disrupting our sleep, which leads to our next section.

● SLEEP

According to the Centers for Disease Control and Prevention (CDC), one-third of Americans don't get the recommended seven to eight hours of sleep each night. Sleep is when our bodies would normally make and circulate cytokines. Without enough deep, restorative sleep, our immune system produces less of the molecules that fight inflammation. Studies have also linked sleep deprivation with lower levels of antibodies and other white blood cells, leaving the body more vulnerable to infection. Adequate sleep, on the other hand, enhances the ability of T cells to go after pathogens. Research has even shown that poor sleep makes the seasonal flu shot less effective.

The field of psychoneuroimmunology studies the relationship between the mind and the immune system. Though the concept may have been dismissed in the not-so-distant past, researchers in this area have identified several pathways through which the brain communicates with the immune system.

• LAUGHTER

Each of us has experienced that immediate rush of mood-boosting endorphins that follows an unrestrained, full-body laugh. In the short-term, that same laugh and the diaphragmatic breathing involved will stimulate our lymphatic system, which produces white blood cells and clears waste from the body, among other functions.

There are long-term benefits to laughing as well. We know that harboring feelings of hostility and resentment are associated with the release of chemicals linked to lowered immunity. As part of a Harvard University study, researchers asked participants to think about an angry memory. Doing so led to a six-hour decrease in the subjects' immunoglobulin A (IgA) levels. These important antibodies are located in the sinuses, lungs, and other respiratory tissues, where they serve as first-line defenders against infection.

Positive thoughts, on the other hand, have been shown to have the opposite effect. By promoting the release of stress-fighting neuropeptides, laughter can boost immunity. Several studies have reported that salivary IgA levels increased in participants who had watched a funny movie. Other groups of researchers have observed dramatic increases in natural killer (NK) cell activity in response to a humorous video.

Need another reason to get frisky with your partner? As it turns out, sex increases antibody production. They actually do studies on this stuff, and the results show fewer sick days for those who are the most sexually active. More specifically, people who had sex once or twice per week had 30% more salivary immunoglobulin A, and those who did the deed less frequently were found to have "significantly" lower IgA levels.

━━━   **THE URBAN BODY FIX**

DIET

This is, perhaps, the most important factor over which you have complete control. What you choose to put in your body will form the foundation of your immune-strengthening protocol.

EAT MORE OF THESE:

1. FRUITS AND VEGETABLES

Not that we need research to convince us of this one, but at least four dozen studies have concluded that a diet rich in fruits and vegetables improves immune function. Here are some of the superstars:

*   **Cruciferous vegetables** (broccoli, cauliflower, kale, cabbage, Brussels sprouts): these are loaded with three compounds—sulforaphane, 3,3-di-indolylmethane, and glucosinolates—that contribute molecules to certain types of lymphocytes in an effort to activate other immune cells. Vegetables in the Brassicaceae family also fight inflammation and they especially like to go after cancer cells. On top of all of that, cruciferous veggies increase levels of detoxifying enzymes in the liver and help to remove heavy metals and other harmful compounds from the body.

* Do some veggies pack more of a punch than others? **Broccoli *sprouts*** provide nearly 100 times more sulforaphane than the mature plant. And scales of nutrient density have consistently ranked **watercress** as the most nutritious vegetable, followed frequently by Chinese broccoli, Swiss chard, and beet greens.

* **Berries and citrus.** This one shouldn't be a tough call either. Aside from boasting hefty doses of the antioxidant vitamin C, all varieties of berries contain health-promoting compounds known as phytochemicals. **Ellagic acid**, for example, is found in pomegranates and strawberries and can actually cause cancer cells to commit suicide in a process called apoptosis. The terpenes in cherries are known to fight viruses. The **anthocyanins** that give blueberries their pigment may also inhibit the ability of the influenza virus to enter human cells. More than 5,000 **phytochemicals** have been identified. The best way to take advantage of these benefits is to consume a broad array of colorful berries. You've heard this advice before: *eat the rainbow!*

* It's long been known that blood levels of vitamin C decrease when our bodies are in a state of stress. Vitamin C plays a crucial role in the activity of natural killer cells and lymphocytes. Dozens of studies have confirmed that higher intakes of vitamin C result in a shortened duration and reduced severity of the common cold and other respiratory infections. The dose used in most research was at least one gram, which is far greater than the government's recommended daily allowance (RDA). A medium orange provides about 100mg. This is an instance where supplementation would be preferable.

* Citrus fruits provide additional health benefits beyond those of vitamin C. The d-limonene found in the peels of **oranges and lemons** has antibacterial properties and has been shown in studies to fight *Streptococcus mutans* and other oral bacteria. **D-limonene** also activates enzymes that prevent DNA damage in cells. Additional research has demonstrated its ability to combat a common fungus linked to skin infections and in one study, d-limonene was even shown to destroy stomach cancer cells. The best way to tap into these benefits is through fresh, cold-pressed juice. The whole lemon or orange, rind and all, can be put through a masticating juicer. Just be sure to buy organic citrus to avoid the toxic, gut-damaging, immune-suppressing chemicals prevalent in commonly used industrial pesticides.

2. FERMENTED FOODS

As discussed previously, the composition and diversity of the microbes in your gut can have a major impact on our immune health.

* This category goes far beyond yogurt. Try adding more **sauerkraut**, **kimchi**, and **pickles** into your diet. German researchers have discovered that the lactic acid bacteria used in the production of these foods leads to the formation of a compound in the gut that attaches to immune cell receptors to help activate our defense system.

* A probiotic supplement can be useful here as a means of repopulating the gut with beneficial bacteria, crowding out pathogenic microbes, and increasing production of antibodies and natural killer cells. Look for a product with at least one billion colony-forming units (CFUs) and multiple strains.

3. ALLIUMS

The same sulfuric compounds that give onions and garlic their strong odor also exert antiviral, antibacterial, antifungal, and antiparasitic properties.

* **Shallots** and **leeks** contain the highest levels of these beneficial compounds and the aging process used to make **black garlic** means it offers more inflammation- and tumor-fighting power in comparison to white garlic. (It also has a much sweeter taste!) **Important**: Cooking destroys many of these compounds, so they are best consumed raw.

4. EXTRA VIRGIN OLIVE OIL (EVOO)

Its benefits go beyond heart health and helps explain the longevity seen among Mediterranean populations. EVOO contains oleocanthal, which has been shown in studies to fight inflammation in the same way as non-steroidal anti-inflammatory drugs (NSAIDs), without all of the side effects. EVOO is also rich in antioxidants that protect our DNA from damage.

- **Important**: The olive oil industry was recently marred by a scandal that called into question the quality of some of the most recognizable brands on the market. An analysis by researchers at the University of California-Davis determined that many producers were cutting their olive oil with cheaper oils. These companies seem to have cleaned up their act after the backlash that ensued but it's still advisable to stick to products tested and certified by one of the following third-party groups: the California Olive Oil Council (COOC), the International Olive Oil Council (IOOC), or the North American Olive Oil Association (NAOOA).

- EVOO has a low smoke point, which means its fatty acids can become damaged and potentially harmful when heated. For this reason, I recommend reserving EVOO for salad dressings or a quick saute. I sometimes add it to my morning smoothie. Trust me, it's undetectable!

5. GOOD FATS

You now know that the omega-6 fatty acids found in many industrial seed oils can promote inflammation in the gut and a depressed immune system. Omega-3's, on the other hand, have been shown to fight inflammation and increase the number of T cells in our immune system.

- To maintain a desirable omega-6:omega-3 ratio, avoid vegetable oils and include more of these healthy fat sources: walnuts, flax seeds, chia seeds, and hemp seeds. As you're likely aware, cold-water fish, such as salmon, sardines, herring, and mackerel provide the highest amounts of these beneficial fats. If you don't consume these foods regularly, you might consider a fish oil or algae-based omega-3 supplement. Quality varies widely and rancid oils will do more harm than good so look for a product with a 5-star rating from the International Fish Oil Standards (IFOS) group. Research has shown that high-DHA fish oil supplements can increase the activity of B cells in the immune system.

- The easiest way to eliminate inflammatory vegetable oils is to cook your own food. Unless otherwise stated on the menu, you can assume that most restaurants are cooking with vegetable oil, most commonly soybean or canola. Knowing this, I actually bring a few fish oil capsules with me when dining out to help shift my 6:3 ratio in the right direction. And if you don't eat processed food, it's unlikely you're consuming much vegetable oil. In your own cooking, opt for avocado oil and macadamia oil when using higher temperatures, as when pan-frying or roasting. Coconut oil is another great option and provides a host of immune-boosting effects thanks to its lauric acid content.

6. GINGER

The benefits of ginger go beyond nausea-prevention and stomach-soothing. Ginger contains the anti-inflammatory compound *gingerol,* and two grams of the herb resulted in "significantly reduced inflammation" among participants at greater risk for colon cancer, as reported in a 2012 article in the *European Journal of Cancer Prevention.* A 2012 study in the *Journal of Ethnopharmacology* reported that 300 micrograms of fresh ginger can trigger cells in our respiratory tract to release antiviral proteins. A separate study in the *Annals of Clinical Microbiology and Antimicrobials* discussed the ability of ginger to fight *E. coli,* including a strain resistant to treatment with antibiotics.

7. HONEY

Compounds in honey restrict the ability of viruses and other pathogens to replicate. Raw honey, in particular, is loaded with antioxidants and is able to inhibit pathogens ranging from *E. coli* and salmonella to staph infections and the bacteria that causes urinary tract infections.

8. MUSHROOMS

They've been used for medicinal purposes for thousands of years and now we have the science to support their immune-boosting power. The benefits come from polysaccharides, most notably beta-glucan. These compounds activate our immune system, but in a balanced way. This is known as immunomodulation. Polysaccharides also stimulate natural killer (NK) cells and favorably alter the microbiota. Mushrooms are particularly aggressive in fighting cancer cells.

They've been used for medicinal purposes for thousands of years and now we have the science to support their immune-boosting power. The benefits come from polysaccharides, most notably beta-glucan. These compounds activate our immune system, but in a balanced way. This is known as immunomodulation. Polysaccharides also stimulate natural killer (NK) cells and favorably alter the microbiota. Mushrooms are particularly aggressive in fighting cancer cells.

There are thousands of varieties of mushrooms but the most well-studied in the area of immune health are shitake, cordyceps, reishi, lion's mane, maitake, and turkey tail. These can be used in soups, stews, and stir-fries and can also be made into teas. Supplements are available in the form of powder or liquid extract. If you go this route, make sure you look for the word "mycelium" on the label.

* Mushrooms that have been exposed to sunlight are a decent source of **vitamin D** but this is not a reliable strategy to obtain a nutrient that is more strongly linked to immune health than most others. In fact, researchers have described that association as "indisputable" and more of them are now calling for government health agencies to strengthen their recommendations for this nutrient. Vitamin D deficiency has been established as a major risk factor for several autoimmune conditions, including multiple sclerosis. Study after study has shown that vitamin D can activate immune cells in the respiratory tract, lowering the risk of the flu and the common cold. Recent studies have suggested a protective effect of vitamin D in COVID-19 patients.

- If you were only going to supplement with one nutrient for immune health, it had better be vitamin D. Most Americans are deficient and there are very few reliable food sources. Unless the largest parts of your body are exposed to the sun for at least 15 minutes several times a week—without sunscreen—you need a supplement. The Vitamin D Council recommends 5,000 International Units per day for most adults.

SLEEP

1. **Bedtime rituals.** If you have a hard time falling and staying asleep, and if you don't wake up feeling rested, this may be indicative of poor sleep *hygiene*, so a new pre-bed protocol may be in order. For starters, be sure to unplug from all electronic devices at least one or two hours before bed. This means putting away all screens, which emit **blue light** and **suppress the body's natural production of melatonin**. If this isn't possible, invest in a pair of blue-light blocking glasses. Felix Gray, Warby Parker, and Uvex each make a good pair, but there are many others. I also recommend downloading **f.lux** on each of your devices. This software can reduce blue light and eye strain. Chamomile tea is a tried-and-true remedy for insomnia.

2. Habit-forming prescription sleep aids should be avoided but many natural alternatives are available. **Valerian**, **passionflower**, and **lemon balm** are quite effective. These herbs affect our brain's receptors for gamma-aminobutyric (GABA), a calm-inducing amino acid. Available in supplement form and as a tea, these herbs produce a mild sedative effect and study results indicate significantly higher measures for sleep quality. Low-dose supplemental melatonin can be used temporarily but, as it is a hormone, long-term use should be avoided.

STRESS REDUCTION

1. The Mindfulness-Based Stress Reduction (MBSR) industry has witnessed a boom in recent years as Americans report feeling more stressed than ever. Scientific support for some of these modalities may be scant but they've been staples of Eastern medicine for centuries and carry little downside. If you've decided that you're not the *meditation* type or if you assume that mindfulness involves sitting still, cross-legged and in solitude and getting spiritual, it's time to open your mind and get up to speed. The Western version of meditation may not resemble much of its origin, but that doesn't make it any less effective. You've got options, even if you assume you're not zen enough:

   * Guided imagery

   * Qi gong

   * Tai chi

   * Yoga

You don't need to attend a retreat to reap the benefits of these techniques. Glo and CorePower are two popular services on-demand yoga classes. Laughter Yoga is now a thing as well.

* **Deep breathing exercises** can lower stress hormones like cortisol and enhance immunity. If the concept of mindfulness is confusing and overwhelming to you and you're not sure where to start, I'd recommend the apps Headspace and Calm. Both offer free programs and a variety of features.

* Stress relief supplements. **Theanine** is my top recommendation here. This is the amino acid responsible for the relaxation benefits associated with tea consumption. **Ashwagandha** is considered an adaptogen, which means it helps your body become more resilient to the effects of stress. It does this, in part, by reducing cortisol levels. **Rhodiola** is another adaptogen that many find helpful in fighting the feeling of burnout associated with chronic stress.

- Aromatherapy. **Lavender** essential oil may have a calming effect when inhaled as a spray or through the use of a diffuser or when applied topically to the skin.

- Recent studies have shown that **pets** can boost the immune system in a way that fights allergies and asthma in children. Apparently, bacteria in a dog's saliva favorably alter our own microbiome. Separately, Swedish researchers found an association between dog ownership and lower mortality. This result supports previous findings demonstrating that simply petting a dog was sufficient to increase one's IgA levels.

- Technology anxiety is a real thing and you'd probably benefit from some digital detox. But, if you're going to stare at a screen anyway, opt for a stress-reliever: Search for a comedy podcast on iTunes or Spotify or follow a funny Instagram meme account.

- Longevity researchers observe several common threads among the longest-living populations on earth. Among them are spending time outdoors, engaging in hobbies or learning new skills, social interaction, and community. These provide a host of mental health benefits, including a sense of belonging, self-worth, fulfillment, motivation, and confidence.

SAUNA

- People in Finland have been using them for generations but only recently has science pinpointed some benefits beyond relaxation. How do the hot temperatures impact immunity? The mechanism is similar to that of exercise: a short-term stressor to which the body responds by increasing the production white blood cells and T cells. In one study, regular sauna users experienced significantly fewer colds, and additional research showed a 30% reduced risk of colds and flu.

FASTING

- Intermittent fasting (IF) is trendy these days, mostly as a means of shedding a few pounds. An extended period without eating leads to a depletion of white blood cells, followed by a corresponding production of new immune cells. IF can also lower inflammation levels in the body and longer fasts of up to 72 hours are associated with increased health benefits, especially among cancer patients.

This chapter isn't meant to be a deep dive into the complexities of the human immune system, the depth and breadth of which can—and has—filled entire volumes. My hope, rather, is that our discussion on immunity will serve as a timely reminder of the privilege *and* the responsibility attached to being in the driver's seat when it comes to our health.

There's not a single tip, strategy, or recommendation referenced above that can guarantee the avoidance of disease. What this template should reveal, however, is the immense power and control we have on an individual level, and through the choices we make each day, to manage risk.

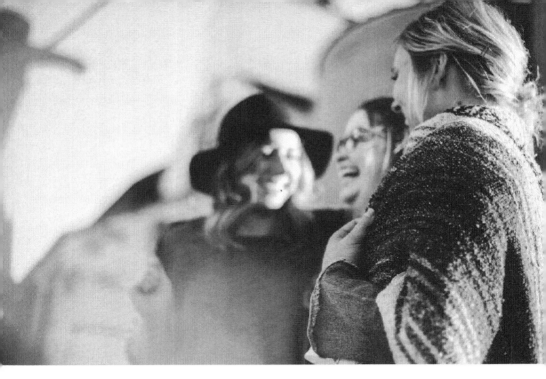

CHAPTER 11

Laugh and Smile a Lot

Imagine a drug that can boost mood, reduce blood pressure, enhance immunity, increase our productivity at work, and make us instantly more attractive to others—all without any side effects and provided free of charge. Would you take it? Well, you don't have to imagine. You can get a dose of it right now, just by conjuring an amusing image or thought. It's actually not a drug at all, but its effects are as powerful as some pharmaceuticals, minus the safety concerns and financial cost.

The simple act of smiling triggers a cascade of events within the body that exert therapeutic physiological and psychological effects, possibly even prolonging our lives. Through similar mechanisms, laughter can also help us heal. This concept was of such interest to researchers in the 1960s that it became a formal field of study—gelotology.

The science behind laughing and smiling provides a compelling case for their inclusion in our natural wellness toolkit. As we review some of the research in this area, you'll recognize some familiar terms. By now you're clear on the interconnectedness of mind and body. You understand that we often react in a physical way based on how we think and feel. And you've seen how certain brain chemicals influence nearly all of our bodily functions. It won't surprise you, then, that these very same neurotransmitters—dopamine, serotonin, GABA—are responsible for the mood-boosting, stress-busting benefits we receive when we smile or laugh. But outside of promoting happiness and a positive outlook, what can these activities do for us? Quite a bit, according to a growing body of research.

In a 2008 study published in the *Journal of Pain*, researchers performed an unpleasant procedure on subjects involving the application of heat. Participants who were told to frown during the experiment reported experiencing more pain than those who smiled or maintained a neutral expression.

In a separate study, this one in 2011, researchers assessed pain tolerance by having subjects hold the bottom position of a wall squat until no longer tolerable or with the application of a wine cooler sleeve frozen to -16°C for up to three minutes. The results of the study demonstrated that pain threshold is significantly higher after laughter.

So what's at play here? Laughter is thought to stimulate the release of endorphins. Yes, the same endorphins released during, exercise, a massage, or chiropractic treatment. Recall that these natural pain-killers can produce an opiate effect in the short-term and may explain the ability of smiling and laughter to relieve aches and pains.

If for no other reason than by providing a distraction, smiling is known to counter psychological and emotional stress. That's a bigger deal than it may sound. A study in *Psychological Science* determined that smiling—even when forced—leads to a lower heart rate in response to hardship or trauma. The College of Family Physicians tells us that a bout of laughter can reduce blood pressure, which helps fight cardiovascular disease.

A study published in 2017 in the *Journal of Dental and Medical Research* found that hemodialysis patients who listened to comedy CDs experienced a decrease in blood pressure. And a comparison study found that laughter through "playful eye contact" and breathing exercises led to a more significant reduction in blood pressure than music therapy; the effect was even more dramatic after a three-month period.

Endothelial dysfunction is another risk factor for heart disease, and laughter seems to help here as well. In a University of Maryland study, researchers measured blood vessel activity in participants after watching either a comedy (*Saturday Night Live*) or drama (*Saving Private Ryan*). Those who watched the comedy had normally functioning blood vessel activity, but blood flow was 35% slower in those who watched the more serious program.

Earlier in the book we discussed the benefits of deep breathing not only in terms of relaxation, but also as a means of delivering adequate oxygen to the lungs and removing stale air. Stress makes our breathing more shallow, resulting in weaker respiratory muscles and making more work for the heart. A prolonged laugh, however, involves a long exhalation, which eliminates residual air. This means more oxygen-rich air for the blood, and increased movement through the respiratory system, which could be beneficial with conditions like asthma or emphysema.

In similar fashion, the act of laughing can stimulate our lymphatic system—the same lymphatic system targeted during massage therapy, as we learned about earlier in the book. Laughter involves movement, "unclogging" lymph and pushing metabolic waste and other toxins through the body for removal.

Many of the other modalities we've highlighted throughout the book have powerful effects on the immune system. Can we put laughter and smiling in that category as well? We certainly can. Through both direct and indirect pathways, each of these activities can bolster our natural defenses.

As previously discussed, chronic emotional and psychological stress makes us more prone to infection. Humor can shut down cortisol production, increase our levels of antibodies, and enhance the function of immune cells.

In a 2015 study published in the Journal of *Alternative and Complementary Medicine*, researchers measured the levels of immunoglobulin (IgA) in the breast milk of postpartum mothers and found that they had increased after laugh therapy. This is significant, as these levels typically decline postpartum.

Research published in 1989 in the *American Journal of Medical Science* revealed significantly increased levels of natural killer (NK) activity in a group of men who had just watched funny videos. Recall that these specialized white blood cells are the first line of defense against viruses and tumor cells.

Cheer and lightheartedness also seems to benefit those with diabetes, one of the most common chronic diseases facing Americans today. Researchers in one study measured blood sugar levels in diabetics after sitting through a dull lecture and then again after watching a comedy. They noted that blood sugar levels were lower in response to the more humorous programming.

We know that bouts of fun can favorably alter brain function, but does that prove beneficial for patients suffering from neurodegenerative disease? Indeed, laugh therapy is increasingly used as an intervention for those with dementia and Parkinson's disease. In fact, an Australian study determined that the effects of this type of therapy are comparable to those of prescription drugs. How? Most likely by calming the agitated state that characterizes many of these conditions—in both patient and caregiver.

Is laughing a form of exercise? Well, it certainly engages the abdominal muscles and will help you burn some extra calories. While there's little scientific research on the much more recent phenomenon known as Laughter Yoga, devotees frequently report improved sleep and diminished pain. These laughter clubs have spread throughout the world and now number in the thousands, including at schools, prisons, and hospitals. In addition to the expected breathing exercises and stretches, Laughter Yoga incorporates silly faces, plenty of eye contact, and optional hugs, all interspersed with sudden bursts of boisterous howling, some on cue and others for absolutely no reason at all.

Fits of laughter involve abdominal contractions, while smiling works your facial muscles, about a dozen in total. They have names like the zygomaticus major and minor, which are responsible for raising the corners of your mouth and the orbicularis oculi, which makes your eyes wrinkle. As with any other type of muscles, these can be strengthened and toned with regular use.

Frowning, on the other hand, uses fewer muscles. Interestingly, botox recipients typically report being happier. Why? Perhaps because the procedure prevents frowning!

We shouldn't need a study to confirm this, but the National Library of Medicine has conducted research showing that people who smile are seen as more likeable. This quality makes it easier to bond with others and increases our self-esteem.

A *Psychology and Aging* study found that we appear younger to others when we smile compared to when pictures of the same person making an angry face are shown.

Observing someone else smile also benefits us. Research has shown that when we look at a smiling face, we feel rewarded. And, unsurprisingly, scientists at the Face Research Laboratory at the University of Aberdeen in Scotland have demonstrated that we're more attracted to people who smile.

Perhaps you've heard that smiling is contagious? When subjects in a Swedish study were shown images depicting various emotions, they automatically imitated the expressions they saw in the pictures, even when being instructed to frown.

According to these "smile researchers," smiling is a means through which we express our emotions. Frowning reflects suppression of our feelings and is associated with negative word choice and memory issues. The conclusion is that trying to silence these emotions causes them to leak into other areas; smiling is how we release those pent-up frustrations.

Economic researchers have long told us that happiness in the workplace leads to greater productivity. By triggering dopamine release, smiling can increase creativity among employees.

Top schools—MIT, Wharton, the London Business School—have all reported benefits to smiling, laughter, and an overall atmosphere of amusement. These include collaboration and engagement. And lower levels of workplace stress usually means less absenteeism.

- Your brain can't tell whether your smile is phony or genuine. If you're down in the dumps, force a smile and eventually smiling will become more habitual.

- Tune out negativity in film, on television, and across social media platforms. Instead, seek out uplifting content.

- If social distancing guidelines have forced the closure of your favorite comedy club, turn to Comedy Central, the many comedy channels on satellite radio, YouTube, Netflix, Hulu, Amazon Prime, or any other streaming service.

- Google "best jokes"or check out the humor section of your local bookstore.

- You're 30 times more likely to laugh when among others than alone. Host a party or game night, even if remotely.

- Fit laughter into your day, as you would exercise or any other appointment. Set aside 10 to 15 minutes to do nothing but laugh.

- Fill your circle with lighthearted and optimistic friends who laugh and smile often.

- Check out the Laughter Online University for helpful ebooks and videos.

- Anticipation of a funny event can be just as powerful. In a 2006 study, men who were told they were going to watch something funny later on, had much higher levels of dopamine and serotonin.

- Get lost in the hilarious memes on someecards.com or spend some time on Will Farrell's Funny Or Die.

- Make faces in the mirror.

- While even a forced smile has benefits, the most authentic will have a more powerful effect. This would be the Duchenne smile, which involves the muscles around the eyes and not just the corners of the mouth. Named after a French neurologist, the Duchenne smile is known to activate different parts of the brain compared to your basic "say cheese" smile. Researchers at the University of California have even proposed that it can predict happiness in marriage decades later!

- Observe and spend time with children. There are many lessons we can learn from kids. They teach us to be more curious, to live in the present, and to try new things. We smile less as we transition from childhood to adulthood. In fact, the average child smiles 400 times each day, compared to just 15 for us grown-ups! We can all benefit from pursuing and then honing a more childlike playfulness.

Nobody likes to be around someone who is always sulking. While we can't control everything that happens to us, we always have the choice to smile. Most situations in life have some underlying "seed" of ridiculousness. Even though it might seem like there's little to laugh about these days, these are the times when we need it the most. Don't question why someone in front of you is laughing so much; question why you're not!

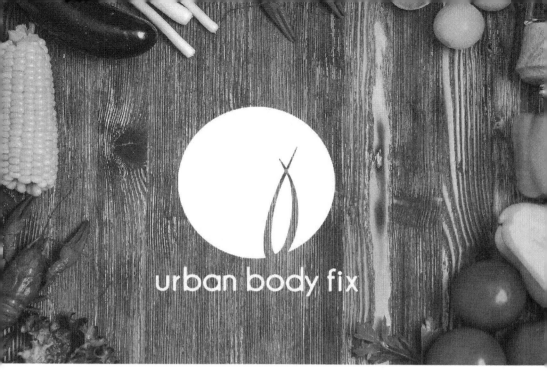

Prescribing Wellness—
The Not-So-Secret Secret to Getting
Everything You Want in Life

In my wildest dreams I never would have imagined the direction my life has taken. By the ripe old age of 47, I have learned quite a bit. I know there's more to come. I embrace that and look forward to the massive shifts that lie ahead. That's the thing: The only constant in life is change. Allowing that change to happen is what makes for a rich life full of surprises and delights.

In this book, I've covered all facets of wellness and how to incorporate them to have a strong and flexible body and mind. So you may ask, what is it all for? I say it's for vibrance. I say it's for adventure. I say it's for fun and passion. This is what you can't measure, but what you feel. We put in the good food, do the best exercise, take the highest quality supplements, and identify the finest practitioners to be our "pit crew"...and then we really get to LIVE. And by living, I mean vibrant living.

When was the last time you thought about all of the things you want to do with this life you've been given? We know it all starts with health because without that, nothing else matters. But when we feel great, we get to do extraordinary things.

Before social media, we often relied on our elders for pearls of wisdom. I may be dating myself, but one such adage—passed down through generations—was the idea that "health is wealth."

Before you dismiss this as another one of those tired clichés or cheesy catchphrases that pop up in your Instafeed (the ones that do more to irritate than inspire), let's consider its original meaning. Whether you attribute this quote to Virgil in 70 BC or Ralph Waldo Emerson in the 1800s, it's likely that wealth in an earlier time wasn't defined exclusively by how much money one had. More precisely, the concept of wealth once encompassed the ability to enjoy that money, to contribute to society, to maintain a social network, and to achieve all-around growth as a person.

Today, though, we often sacrifice our health in the quest for affluence and abundance. In a 2018 study in the journal *Nature Human Behavior*, greater income was "associated with reduced life satisfaction and a lower level of well-being." Health is quickly becoming an outdated term. It's not possible to quantify health by any single metric and there's no one-size-fits-all standard for it. If you've made it to this point in the book, you know I prefer the term *wellness*. You also know that life satisfaction and well-being are two major components of the concept of wellness. So if having more stuff means less happiness, are we really healthy? Or well?

According to a Harvard Business Review analysis, wealth can also be isolating. When we achieve it, the researchers concluded, we become more suspicious of others and we tend to cut ourselves off from colleagues, friends, and even family. We know from previous studies that our connections to others—not material objects—bring us the most joy and satisfaction in life.

Having time to engage, to love, and to experience gratitude also rank highly among respondents in these surveys. These are also key components of wellness.

This goes without saying, but you can have all the money in the world and still be sick in mind, body, or spirit. Could you enjoy even a penny of it, then? On the other hand, you can still be happy if you're healthy. Ideally, of course, you'd have both. And that's the beauty of the *Urban Body Fix*: In a healthy state you have a better shot at attaining wealth and success. Good health allows you to pursue happiness, but without it, life stops or becomes more difficult. Poor health is a barrier, and depending on the nature of the health issue, it can nag in a way that's merely bothersome or it can dominate and consume you. Poor health is always there—but so is vibrant wellness.

When you are well, you have the freedom and flexibility to focus on the other most important things in your life: family, friends, passions, and purpose—all without worry or distraction. Wellness—in each of its facets—provides the foundation from which to pursue your passions and interests, to enjoy them and experience them more fully and deeply. You need vigor and energy to be present in those other areas, and not the kind you get from coffee, energy drinks, or other stimulants. With total wellness, you're humming along with a smooth, steady, motivating clarity. Fewer doctors and meds = more wealth. The longer you're healthy, the longer you can continue to gain wealth.

In writing this book, I have tried hard to go beyond theory, to provide specific action steps addressing all facets of our health, an idea that extends far beyond our fixation with the physical realm to also include mental, emotional, and spiritual well-being. This new paradigm of health—wellness—acknowledges that most illness is the result of poor lifestyle choices that we have the power and responsibility to change. Maybe these concepts weren't priorities for you in the past (they weren't always for me) and the reality is that we have all done some damage to our health before we decided—in our own way and for our own reasons—to right the ship. Whenever, wherever, or however that seed was unearthed, the soil now must be cultivated and the plant needs nourishment to bear fruit, to flourish, and to thrive.

No matter where you are in that process, you'll experience setbacks, but only when you lose sight of our themes of balance and moderation. Perhaps you hit the gym daily but you're constantly amped up and make no time for relaxation. Or maybe you're a devout yogi but you succumb to the health halo effect of vegan cookies and plant-based ice cream and your diet contains very few fruits and vegetables.

Balance and moderation represent a harmony measured not in terms of pounds or calories but instead gauged by how we persevere in the face of the bumps and bruises on our road to fulfillment throughout life and in old age. To design the life we want, our wellness toolkit needs one final addition: resilience. If you get sick, resilience allows you to fight. When starting a weight-loss plan, resilience keeps you on track. In business, resilience helps you weather and adapt to disruptions.

Recall our pillars of wellness from Chapter 1. When we allow ourselves to become overwhelmed, one or more of these areas will be neglected. Strive for small changes and targeted choices and these will accumulate, providing momentum to propel you forward on your journey. After all, what is the best way to eat an elephant? One bite at a time! Be patient and put yourself first once in a while. It's not selfish. Those who rely on you will benefit from a more vibrant you. You only get one mind and one body and you can't buy new ones. Like wealth, we don't realize the value of wellness until we've lost it.

The power of taking responsibility for my own health has led me to unimaginable places. Most importantly is that it provides clarity and vigor. We make choices yearly, monthly, weekly, hourly and minute to minute. These choices shape who we are. Not every choice is the best one, but it gets you to where you need to be in life. When you have good health you have clear thinking and are able to navigate life more seamlessly. My journey through wellness propelled me to build the *Urban Body Fix* brand and beyond. My journey through wellness has allowed me to pursue my passions. One of those passions was to be a Broadway producer and I'm happy to say I've achieved that goal, even earning a Tony Award along the way. Whatever wild dream you may have, chase it! It just might come true. I have a family and a life that I love. I wish that for every person on the planet who wants a vibrant life.

Get your health handled.

The wealth will follow, and then the world will be teeming with possibilities.

References

─────── **CHAPTER 1**

International Communication Association. "Feelings of loneliness, depression linked to binge-watching television." ScienceDaily. ScienceDaily, 29 January 2015.

Dell'Osso, Liliana, Abelli, Marianna, Carpita, Barbara, Pini, Stefano, Castellini, Giovanni, Carmassi, Claudia, and Ricca, Valdo. Historical evolution of the concept of anorexia nervosa and relationships with orthorexia nervosa, autism, and obsessive–compulsive spectrum. *Neuropsychiatr Dis Treat.* 2016; 12: 1651–1660.

Jane Ogden et al. Distraction, restrained eating and disinhibition: An experimental study of food intake and the impact of 'eating on the go'. *Journal of Health Psychology Ogden*, August 2015. DOI: 10.1177/1359105315595119

Chen Y, Lin YC, Zimmerman CA, Essner RA, Knight ZA. Hunger neurons drive feeding through a sustained, positive reinforcement signal. *Elife.* 2016;5:e18640. Published 2016 Aug 24. doi:10.7554/eLife.18640.

─────── **CHAPTER 2**

Center for Disease Control and Prevention (CDC), National Center for Health Statistics, Obesity and Overweight

Center for Disease Control and Prevention (CDC) Press Release, July, 18, 2017

American Heart Association (AHA), Heart Disease and Stroke Statistics-2019 At-a-Glance

The US Burden of Disease Collaborators. The State of US Health, 1990-2016: Burden of Diseases, Injuries, and Risk Factors Among US States. JAMA. 2018;319(14):1444–1472. doi:10.1001/jama.2018.0158

Weingarten HP, Elston D. Food cravings in a college population. Appetite. 1991;17(3):167-175. doi:10.1016/0195-6663(91)90019-0

Hill AJ, Weaver CF, Blundell JE. Food craving, dietary restraint and mood. Appetite. 1991;17(3):187-197. doi:10.1016/0195-6663(91)90021-j

Rogers PJ, Smit HJ. Food craving and food "addiction": a critical review of the evidence from a biopsychosocial perspective. Pharmacol Biochem Behav. 2000;66(1):3-14. doi:10.1016/s0091-3057(00)00197-0

Weingarten HP, Elston D. The phenomenology of food cravings. Appetite. 1990;15(3):231-246. doi:10.1016/0195-6663(90)90023-2

Macedo DM, Diez-Garcia RW. Sweet craving and ghrelin and leptin levels in women during stress. Appetite. 2014;80:264-270. doi:10.1016/j.appet.2014.05.031

Taheri, Shahrad, Lin, Ling, Austin, Diane, Young, Terry, and Emmanuel Mignot, Emmanuel: Short Sleep Duration Is Associated with Reduced Leptin, Elevated Ghrelin, and Increased Body Mass Index. *PLoS Med.* 2004 Dec; 1(3): e62.x

Hormes, Julia M., Niemiec, Martha A.: Does culture create craving? Evidence from the case of menstrual chocolate craving. *PLoS Med.* 2017 Jul 19

Martin, C.K., Rosenbaum, D., Han, H., Geiselman, P., Wyatt, H., Hill, J., Brill, C., Bailer, Miller, B.V. III, Stein, R., Klein, S., and Foster, Gard D.: Change in food cravings, food preferences, and appetite during a low-carbohydrate and low-fat diet. *Obesity* (Silver Spring). 2011 Oct; 19(10): 1963–1970.

Yang, Qing. Gain weight by "going diet?" Artificial sweeteners and the neurobiology of sugar cravings. *Yale J Biol Med.* 2010 Jun; 83(2): 101–108.

Blackwell, Debra, L. and Clarke, Tainya C. State Variation in Meeting the 2008 Federal Guidelines for Both Aerobic and Muscle-strengthening Activities Through Leisure-time Physical Activity Among Adults Aged 18–64: United States, 2010– 2015. *National Health Statistics Reports*, Number 112. 2018 Jun 28.

Guthold, Regina, PhD, Stevens, Gretchen A. DSc, Leanne M., MSc, Prof Fiona C Bull, Fiona C.,PhD. Worldwide trends in insufficient physical activity from 2001 to 2016: a pooled analysis of 358 population-based surveys with 1·9 million participants. *The Lancet Global Health*, Volume 6, Issue 10 2018: Oct 1, E1077-E1086.

Meckel Y, Eliakim A, Seraev M, et al. The effect of a brief sprint interval exercise on growth factors and inflammatory mediators. J Strength Cond Res. 2009;23(1):225-230. doi:10.1519/JSC.0b013e3181876a9a

Bhammar DM, Angadi SS, Gaesser GA. Effects of fractionized and continuous exercise on 24-h ambulatory blood pressure. Med Sci Sports Exerc. 2012;44(12):2270-2276. doi:10.1249/MSS.0b013e3182663117

Holman RM, Carson V, Janssen I. Does the fractionalization of daily physical activity (sporadic vs. bouts) impact cardiometabolic risk factors in children and youth?. PLoS One. 2011;6(10):e25733. doi:10.1371/journal.pone.0025733

Quinn TJ, Klooster JR, Kenefick RW. Two short, daily activity bouts vs. one long bout: are health and fitness improvements similar over twelve and twenty-four weeks?. J Strength Cond Res. 2006;20(1):130-135. doi:10.1519/R-16394.1

Zhang, Jingwen PhD, Brackbill, Devon PhD, Yang, Sijia MA, Becker, Joshua MA, Herbert, Natalie MA, Damon, Centola PhD. Support or competition? How online social networks increase physical activity: A randomized controlled trial. *Preventive Medicine Reports* Volume 4, December 2016, Pages 453-458.

Ekelund, Ulf, Tarp, Jakob,Steene-Johannessen, Jostein, Hansen, Bjorge H., Jefferis, Barbara, Fagerland, Morten W., Whincup, Peter, Diaz, Keith M., Hooker, Steven P., Chernofsky, Ariel, Larson, Martin G., Spartano, Nicole, Vasan, Ramachandran S.,Dohrn, Ing-Mari, Hagströmer, Maria, Edwardson, Charlotte, Yates, Thomas, Shiroma, Eric, Anderssen, Sigmund A.,Lee, I-Min. Dose-response associations between accelerometry measured physical activity and sedentary time and all cause mortality: systematic review and harmonised meta-analysis. *BMJ* 2019 Aug; 366 doi: https://doi.org/10.1136/bmj.l4570

CHAPTER 5

Rapaport MH, Schettler P, Larson ER, et al. Acute Swedish Massage Monotherapy Successfully Remediates Symptoms of Generalized Anxiety Disorder: A Proof-of-Concept, Randomized Controlled Study. J Clin Psychiatry. 2016;77(7):e883-e891. doi:10.4088/JCP.15m10151

Field, Tiffany, Hernandez-Reif, Maria, Diego, Miguel, Schanberg, Saul, Kuhn, Cynthia. Cortisol Decreases and Serotonin and Dopamine Increase Following Massage Therapy.
International Journal of Neuroscience. Volume 115, 2005 - Issue 10.

Mehl-Madrona, Lewis MD, PhD, Kligler, Benjamin MD, MPH, Silverman, Shoshana MSW, Lynton, Holly BS, Merrell, Woodson, MD. The Impact of Acupuncture and Craniosacral Therapy Interventions on Clinical Outcomes in Adults With Asthma. *Explore.* Volume 3, Issue 1, January 2007, Pages 28-36.

Li, Yan-hui, Wang, Feng-yun, Feng, Chun-qing, Yang, Xia-feng, and Sun, Yi-hua. Massage Therapy for Fibromyalgia: A Systematic Review and Meta-Analysis of Randomized Controlled Trials. PLoS One. 2014; 9(2): e89304.

Raviv, Gil, Shefi, Shai, Nizani, Dalia, Achorin, Anat. Effect of craniosacral therapy on lower urinary tract signs and symptoms in multiple sclerosis. *Complementary Therapies in Clinical Practice.* Volume 15, Issue 2, May 2009, Pages 72-75.

Effect of massage in postmenopausal women with insomnia – A pilot study. *Clinics* (Sao Paulo). 2011 Feb; 66(2): 343–346.

Zainal Zainuddin, Zainal, Newton, Mike, Sacco, Paul and Kazunori Nosaka, Kazunori. Effects of Massage on Delayed-Onset Muscle Soreness, Swelling, and Recovery of Muscle Function. *J Athl Train*. 2005 Jul-Sep; 40(3): 174–180.

Preyde M. Effectiveness of massage therapy for subacute low-back pain: a randomized controlled trial. *CMAJ*. 2000;162(13):1815-1820.

Lipton SA. Prevention of classic migraine headache by digital massage of the superficial temporal arteries during visual aura. *Ann Neurol*. 1986;19(5):515-516. doi:10.1002/ana.410190521.

Quinn, Christopher DC, Chandler, Clint BS, and Moraska, Albert PhD. Massage Therapy and Frequency of Chronic Tension Headaches. *Am J Public Health*. 2002 October; 92(10): 1657–1661.

Field T, Hernandez-Reif M, Seligman S, et al. Juvenile rheumatoid arthritis: benefits from massage therapy. *J Pediatr Psychol*. 1997;22(5):607-617. doi:10.1093/jpepsy/22.5.607

Kinkead B, Schettler PJ, Larson ER, et al. Massage therapy decreases cancer-related fatigue: Results from a randomized early phase trial. *Cancer*. 2018;124(3):546-554. doi:10.1002/cncr.31064

Sun, Nuo, Youle, Richard J., and Finkel, Toren. The Mitochondrial Basis of Aging. *Mol Cell*. 2016 Mar 3; 61(5): 654–666.

Hernandez-Reif M, Field T, Ironson G, et al. Natural killer cells and lymphocytes increase in women with breast cancer following massage therapy. *Int J Neurosci*. 2005;115(4):495-510. doi:10.1080/00207450590523080

Green, Victoria L., Alexandropoulou, Afroditi, Walker, Mary B., Walker, Andrew A., Sharp, Donald M., Walker, Leslie G., and Greenman, John. Alterations in the Th1/Th2 balance in breast cancer patients using reflexology and scalp massage. *Exp Ther Med*. 2010 Jan-Feb; 1(1): 97–108.

Crane, Justin D., Ogborn, Daniel I., Cupido, Colleen, Melov, Simon, Hubbard, Alan, Bourgeois,, Jacqueline M., Tarnopolsky, Mark A. Massage Therapy Attenuates Inflammatory Signaling After Exercise-Induced Muscle Damage. *Science Translational Medicine*. 01 Feb 2012 : 119RA13

CHAPTER 6

Kunst, Alexander. U.S. adults with positive view on complementary and alternative medicine 2017. *Statista*. Sep 3, 2019.

Salehi, Alireza MD, MPH, PhD, Hashemi, Neda MSc, Hadi Imanieh, Mohammad MD, and Saber, Mahboobeh MD. Chiropractic: Is it Efficient in Treatment of Diseases? Review of Systematic Reviews. *Int J Community Based Nurs Midwifery*. 2015 Oct; 3(4): 244–254.

Dailey, Dana L., Rakel, Barbara A., Vance, Carol GT, Liebano, Richard E., Anand, Amrit S., Bush, Heather M., Lee, Kyoung S., Lee, Jennifer E., and Sluka, Kathleen A. Transcutaneous Electrical Nerve Stimulation (TENS) reduces pain, fatigue, and hyperalgesia while restoring central inhibition in primary fibromyalgia. *Pain*. 2013 Nov; 154(11): 2554–2562

Vickers, Andrew J., Vertosick, Emily A., Lewith, George, Claudia M. Witt, Claudia M., Linde, Klaus. Acupuncture for Chronic Pain: Update of an Individual Patient Data Meta-Analysis. *Journal of Pain*. Volume 19, Issue 5, P455-474, May 01, 2018.

Corbett MS, Rice SJ, Madurasinghe V, et al. Acupuncture and other physical treatments for the relief of pain due to osteoarthritis of the knee: network meta-analysis. *Osteoarthritis Cartilage*. 2013;21(9):1290-1298. doi:10.1016/j. joca.2013.05.007.

Dong W, Goost H, Lin XB, et al. Treatments for shoulder impingement syndrome: a PRISMA systematic review and network meta-analysis [published correction appears in Medicine (Baltimore). 2016 Jun 10;95(23):e96d5]. Medicine (Baltimore). 2015;94(10):e510. doi:10.1097/MD.0000000000000510

Lewis RA, Williams NH, Sutton AJ, et al. Comparative clinical effectiveness of management strategies for sciatica: systematic review and network meta-analyses. *Spine J*. 2015;15(6):1461-1477. doi:10.1016/j.spinee.2013.08.049

Vitale, Anne T. MSN, APRN, BC; O'Connor, Priscilla C. PhD, APRN, BC The Effect of Reiki on Pain and Anxiety in Women With Abdominal Hysterectomies: A Quasi-experimental Pilot Study, *Holistic Nursing Practice*: November-December 2006 - Volume 20 - Issue 6 - p 263-272.

Fleisher KA, Mackenzie ER, Frankel ES, Seluzicki C, Casarett D, Mao JJ. Integrative Reiki for cancer patients: a program evaluation. *Integr Cancer Ther*. 2014;13(1):62-67. doi:10.1177/1534735413503547.

Bowden, Deborah, Goddard, Lorna, Gruzelier, John. "A Randomised Controlled Single-Blind Trial of the Efficacy of Reiki at Benefitting Mood and Well-Being", Evidence-Based Complementary and Alternative Medicine, vol. 2011, Article ID 381862, 8pages, 2011. https://doi.org/10.1155/2011/381862.

Jahantiqh F, Abdollahimohammad A, Firouzkouhi M, Ebrahiminejad V. Effects of Reiki Versus Physiotherapy on Relieving Lower Back Pain and Improving Activities Daily Living of Patients With Intervertebral Disc Hernia. *J Evid Based Integr Med*. 2018;23:2515690X18762745. doi:10.1177/2515690X18762745.

Kirsch, Irving, Montgomery, Guy, Sapirstein, Guy. Hypnosis as an adjunct to cognitive-behavioral psychotherapy: A meta-analysis. *Journal of Consulting and Clinical Psychology*, Vol 63(2), Apr 1995, 214-220.

Accardi, M.C., Milling, L.S. The effectiveness of hypnosis for reducing procedure-related pain in children and adolescents: a comprehensive methodological review. *J Behav Med* 32, 328–339 (2009). https://doi.org/10.1007/s10865-009-9207-6.

Maxym, Maya, "Hypnosis for Relief of Pain and Anxiety in Children Receiving Intravenous Lines in the Pediatric Emergency Department" (2008). *Yale Medicine Thesis Digital Library.* 355. http://elischolar.library.yale.edu/ymtdl/355.

Häuser, Winfried PD Dr., Hagl, Maria, Dr. phil. Dipl.-Psych., Albrecht Schmierer, Albrecht, Dr., and Hansen, Emil. Prof.The Efficacy, Safety and Applications of Medical Hypnosis. *Dtsch Arztebl Int.* 2016 Apr; 113(17): 289–296.

Landolt, Alison S., Milling, Leonard S. The efficacy of hypnosis as an intervention for labor and delivery pain: A comprehensive methodological review. *Clinical Psychology Review.* Volume 31, Issue 6, August 2011, Pages 1022-1031.

Timothy P. Carmody, Carol Duncan, Joel A. Simon, Sharon Solkowitz, Joy Huggins, Sharon Lee, Kevin Delucchi, Hypnosis for Smoking Cessation: A Randomized Trial, *Nicotine & Tobacco Research*, Volume 10, Issue 5, May 2008, Pages 811–818, https://doi.org/10.1080/14622200802023833.

J.H. Gruzelier (2002) A Review of the Impact of Hypnosis, Relaxation, Guided Imagery and Individual Differences on Aspects of Immunity and Health, *The International Journal on the Biology of Stress*, 5:2, 147-163, DOI: 10.1080/10253890290027877

CHAPTER 7

APA Stress in America™ Survey: US at 'Lowest Point We Can Remember;' Future of Nation Most Commonly Reported Source of Stress. *American Psychological Association.* November 1, 2017.

Luders, Eileen, Cherbuin, Nicolas, and Gaser, Christian. Estimating brain age using high-resolution pattern recognition: Younger brains in long-term meditation practitioners. *NeuroImage.* 134 (2016) 508-513.

Greenberg, Jonathan, Reiner, Keren, Meiran, Nachshon. "Mind the Trap": Mindfulness Practice Reduces Cognitive Rigidity. *PLOS ONE*. May 15, 2012. https://doi.org/10.1371/journal.pone.0036206.

Bhasin MK, Denninger JW, Huffman JC, et al. Specific Transcriptome Changes Associated with Blood Pressure Reduction in Hypertensive Patients After Relaxation Response Training. *J Altern Complement Med.* 2018;24(5):486-504. doi:10.1089/acm.2017.0053.

Rosenkranz MA, Davidson RJ, Maccoon DG, Sheridan JF, Kalin NH, Lutz A. A comparison of mindfulness-based stress reduction and an active control in modulation of neurogenic inflammation. *Brain Behav Immun.* 2013;27(1):174-184. doi:10.1016/j.bbi.2012.10.013.

Taren, Adrienne A., Gianaros, Peter J., Greco, Carol M., Lindsay, Emily K., Fairgrieve, April, Warren Brown, Kirk,Rosen, Rhonda K., Ferris, Jennifer L., Julson, Erica, Marsland, Anna L., Bursley, James K., Ramsburg, Jared, and Creswel, J. David. lMindfulness meditation training alters stress-related amygdala resting state functional connectivity: a randomized controlled trial. *Soc Cogn Affect Neurosci.* 2015 Dec; 10(12): 1758–1768.

Weng, Helen Y., Fox, Andrew S., Shackman, Alexander J., Stodola, Diane E., Caldwell, Jessica Z.K., Olson, Matthew C., Rogers, Gregory M., and Davidson, Richard J. Compassion training alters altruism and neural responses to suffering. *Psychol Sci.* 2013 Jul 1; 24(7): 1171–1180.

Kozasa EH, Tanaka LH, Monson C, Little S, Leao FC, Peres MP. The effects of meditation-based interventions on the treatment of fibromyalgia. *Curr Pain Headache Rep.* 2012;16(5):383-387. doi:10.1007/s11916-012-0285-8.

Speca, Michael PsyD; Carlson, Linda E. PhD; Goodey, Eileen MSW; Angen, Maureen PhD A Randomized, Wait-List Controlled Clinical Trial: The Effect of a Mindfulness Meditation-Based Stress Reduction Program on Mood and Symptoms of Stress in Cancer Outpatients, *Psychosomatic Medicine*: September-October 2000 - Volume 62 - Issue 5 - p 613-622.

Carmody, James and Baer, Ruth. Relationships between mindfulness practice and levels of mindfulness, medical and psychological symptoms and well-being in a mindfulness-based stress reduction program. March 2008 *Journal of Behavioral Medicine* 31(1):23-33.

Martires J, Zeidler M. The value of mindfulness meditation in the treatment of insomnia. *Curr Opin Pulm Med.* 2015;21(6):547-552. doi:10.1097/MCP.0000000000000207.

Brewer JA, Mallik S, Babuscio TA, et al. Mindfulness training for smoking cessation: results from a randomized controlled trial. *Drug Alcohol Depend.* 2011;119(1-2):72-80. doi:10.1016/j.drugalcdep.2011.05.027.

▬▬▬▬▬   **CHAPTER 8**

Riley, Alex. Why vitamin pills don't work, and may be bad for you. BBC.com. 2016: Dec 8.

Salem, Tala. Study: Vitamin Supplements Don't Provide Health Benefits. usnews. com. 2018: May 29.

Pawlowski, A. Vitamin pills and supplements aren't helping most people, doctors say. Today.com. 2018: Feb 8.

Haspel, Tamar. Most dietary supplements don't do anything. Why do we spend $35 billion a year on them? Washingtonpost.com. 2020: Jan 27.

Kappeler, D., Heimbeck, I., Herpich, C. et al. Higher bioavailability of magnesium citrate as compared to magnesium oxide shown by evaluation of urinary excretion and serum levels after single-dose administration in a randomized cross-over study. *BMC Nutr* 3, 7 (2017). https://doi.org/10.1186/s40795-016-0121-3.

Cardenas E, Ghosh R. Vitamin E: a dark horse at the crossroad of cancer management. *Biochem Pharmacol.* 2013;86(7):845-852. doi:10.1016/j.bcp.2013.07.018

Oregon State University. "Study Finds Huge Variability In Vitamin E Absorption." ScienceDaily. ScienceDaily, 16 January 2004. <www.sciencedaily.com/releases/2004/01/040116073557.html>.

Wright ME, Lawson KA, Weinstein SJ, et al. Higher baseline serum concentrations of vitamin E are associated with lower total and cause-specific mortality in the Alpha-Tocopherol, Beta-Carotene Cancer Prevention Study. *Am J Clin Nutr*. 2006;84(5):1200-1207. doi:10.1093/ajcn/84.5.1200

Shieh A, Chun RF, Ma C, et al. Effects of High-Dose Vitamin D2 Versus D3 on Total and Free 25-Hydroxyvitamin D and Markers of Calcium Balance. *J Clin Endocrinol Metab*. 2016;101(8):3070-3078. doi:10.1210/jc.2016-1871

Armas LA, Hollis BW, Heaney RP. Vitamin D2 is much less effective than vitamin D3 in humans. *J Clin Endocrinol Metab*. 2004;89(11):5387-5391. doi:10.1210/jc.2004-0360

Forrest KY, Stuhldreher WL. Prevalence and correlates of vitamin D deficiency in US adults. *Nutr Res*. 2011;31(1):48-54. doi:10.1016/j.nutres.2010.12.001

Gerster H. Can adults adequately convert alpha-linolenic acid (18:3n-3) to eicosapentaenoic acid (20:5n-3) and docosahexaenoic acid (22:6n-3)?. *Int J Vitam Nutr Res*. 1998;68(3):159-173.

Burr ML, Fehily AM, Gilbert JF, et al. Effects of changes in fat, fish, and fibre intakes on death and myocardial reinfarction: diet and reinfarction trial (DART). *Lancet*. 1989;2(8666):757-761. doi:10.1016/s0140-6736(89)90828-3

Yokoyama M, Origasa H, Matsuzaki M, et al. Effects of eicosapentaenoic acid on major coronary events in hypercholesterolaemic patients (JELIS): a randomised open-label, blinded endpoint analysis [published correction appears in Lancet. 2007 Jul 21;370(9583):220]. *Lancet*. 2007;369(9567):1090-1098. doi:10.1016/S0140-6736(07)60527-3

ORIGIN Trial Investigators, Bosch J, Gerstein HC, et al. n-3 fatty acids and cardiovascular outcomes in patients with dysglycemia. *N Engl J Med*. 2012;367(4):309-318. doi:10.1056/NEJMoa1203859

Lim GP, Calon F, Morihara T, et al. A diet enriched with the omega-3 fatty acid docosahexaenoic acid reduces amyloid burden in an aged Alzheimer mouse model. *J Neurosci.* 2005;25(12):3032-3040. doi:10.1523/JNEUROSCI.4225-04.2005

Yelland LN, Gajewski BJ, Colombo J, Gibson RA, Makrides M, Carlson SE. Predicting the effect of maternal docosahexaenoic acid (DHA) supplementation to reduce early preterm birth in Australia and the United States using results of within country randomized controlled trials. *Prostaglandins Leukot Essent Fatty Acids.* 2016;112:44-49. doi:10.1016/j.plefa.2016.08.007

von Schacky C. A review of omega-3 ethyl esters for cardiovascular prevention and treatment of increased blood triglyceride levels. *Vasc Health Risk Manag.* 2006;2(3):251-262. doi:10.2147/vhrm.2006.2.3.251

Lawson LD, Hughes BG. Human absorption of fish oil fatty acids as triacylglycerols, free acids, or ethyl esters. *Biochem Biophys Res Commun.* 1988;152(1):328-335. doi:10.1016/s0006-291x(88)80718-6v

Reis GJ, Silverman DI, Boucher TM, et al. Effects of two types of fish oil supplements on serum lipids and plasma phospholipid fatty acids in coronary artery disease. *Am J Cardiol.* 1990;66(17):1171-1175. doi:10.1016/0002-9149(90)91093-l

Hansen JB, Olsen JO, Wilsgård L, Lyngmo V, Svensson B. Comparative effects of prolonged intake of highly purified fish oils as ethyl ester or triglyceride on lipids, haemostasis and platelet function in normolipaemic men. *Eur J Clin Nutr.* 1993;47(7):497-507.

Kelly M. Adams, W. Scott Butsch, Martin Kohlmeier, "The State of Nutrition Education at US Medical Schools", *Journal of Biomedical Education*, vol. 2015, Article ID 357627, 7 pages, 2015. https://doi.org/10.1155/2015/357627.

Radlicz, Chris. A Time for Change: Nutrition Education in Medicine. American Society for Nutrition online article. 2017: Dec 4. https://nutrition.org/a-time-for-change-nutrition-education-in-medicine/.

Glauser W. Pharma influence widespread at medical schools: study. *CMAJ*. 2013;185(13):1121-1122. doi:10.1503/cmaj.109-4563

Neel, Joe. Medical Schools and Drug Firm Dollars.npr.com. 2005: Jun 9.

Angell, Marcia. Drug Companies and Medicine: What Money Can Buy. Harvard Medical School lecture. 2009: Dec 10.

Keys T, Ryan MH, Dobie S, Satin D, Evans DV. Premedical Student Exposure to Pharmaceutical Marketing: Too Much, Too Soon? Fam Med. 2019;51(9):722-727. https://doi.org/10.22454/FamMed.2019.360469.

Austad KE, Avorn J, Kesselheim AS. Medical students' exposure to and attitudes about the pharmaceutical industry: a systematic review. PLoS Med. 2011;8(5):e1001037. doi:10.1371/journal.pmed.1001037

Ahluwalia N, Dwyer J, Terry A, Moshfegh A, Johnson C. Update on NHANES Dietary Data: Focus on Collection, Release, Analytical Considerations, and Uses to Inform Public Policy. Adv Nutr. 2016;7(1):121-134. Published 2016 Jan 15. doi:10.3945/an.115.009258

Bird JK, Murphy RA, Ciappio ED, McBurney MI. Risk of Deficiency in Multiple Concurrent Micronutrients in Children and Adults in the United States. Nutrients. 2017;9(7):655. Published 2017 Jun 24. doi:10.3390/nu9070655

CHAPTER 9

Fialho A, Fialho A, Kochhar G, Schenone AL, Thota P, McCullough AJ, Shen B. Association Between Small Intestinal Bacterial Overgrowth by Glucose Breath Test and Coronary Artery Disease. *Dig Dis Sci*. 2018 Feb;63(2):412-421. doi: 10.1007/s10620-017-4828-z. Epub 2017 Nov 6. PMID: 29110161.

Khan A, Dawoud H, Malinski T. Nanomedical studies of the restoration of nitric oxide/peroxynitrite balance in dysfunctional endothelium by 1,25-dihydroxy vitamin D3 – clinical implications for cardiovascular diseases. Int J Nanomedicine. 2018;13:455-466

Yin K, Agrawal DK. Vitamin D and inflammatory diseases. J Inflamm Res. 2014;7:69-87. Published 2014 May 29. doi:10.2147/JIR.S63898

Min B. Effects of vitamin d on blood pressure and endothelial function. Korean J Physiol Pharmacol. 2013;17(5):385-392. doi:10.4196/kjpp.2013.17.5.385

Zozina VI, Covantev S, Goroshko OA, Krasnykh LM, Kukes VG. Coenzyme Q10 in Cardiovascular and Metabolic Diseases: Current State of the Problem. Curr Cardiol Rev. 2018;14(3):164-174. doi:10.2174/1573403X14666180416115428

Montenero AS, Mollichelli N, Zumbo F, et al. Helicobacter pylori and atrial fibrillation: a possible pathogenic link. Heart. 2005;91(7):960-961. doi:10.1136/hrt.2004.036681

Yan J, She Q, Zhang Y, Cui C, Zhang G. The Association between Arrhythmia and Helicobacter pylori Infection: A Meta-Analysis of Case-Control Studies. Int J Environ Res Public Health. 2016;13(11):1139. Published 2016 Nov 16. doi:10.3390/ijerph13111139

Bhattacharyya A, Chattopadhyay R, Mitra S, Crowe SE. Oxidative stress: an essential factor in the pathogenesis of gastrointestinal mucosal diseases. Physiol Rev. 2014;94(2):329-354. doi:10.1152/physrev.00040.2012

Fahey JW, Stephenson KK, Wallace AJ. Dietary amelioration of Helicobacter infection. Nutr Res. 2015;35(6):461-473. doi:10.1016/j.nutres.2015.03.001

Haristoy X, Angioi-Duprez K, Duprez A, Lozniewski A. Efficacy of sulforaphane in eradicating Helicobacter pylori in human gastric xenografts implanted in nude mice. Antimicrob Agents Chemother. 2003;47(12):3982-3984. doi:10.1128/aac.47.12.3982-3984.2003

Khoder G, Al-Menhali AA, Al-Yassir F, Karam SM. Potential role of probiotics in the management of gastric ulcer. Exp Ther Med. 2016;12(1):3-17. doi:10.3892/etm.2016.3293

Lin YT, Kwon YI, Labbe RG, Shetty K. Inhibition of Helicobacter pylori and associated urease by oregano and cranberry phytochemical synergies. Appl Environ Microbiol. 2005;71(12):8558-8564. doi:10.1128/AEM.71.12.8558-8564.2005

Janeiro MH, Ramírez MJ, Milagro FI, Martínez JA, Solas M. Implication of Trimethylamine N-Oxide (TMAO) in Disease: Potential Biomarker or New Therapeutic Target. Nutrients. 2018;10(10):1398. Published 2018 Oct 1. doi:10.3390/nu10101398

Chen ML, Yi L, Zhang Y, et al. Resveratrol Attenuates Trimethylamine-N-Oxide (TMAO)-Induced Atherosclerosis by Regulating TMAO Synthesis and Bile Acid Metabolism via Remodeling of the Gut Microbiota. mBio. 2016;7(2):e02210-e2215. Published 2016 Apr 5. doi:10.1128/mBio.02210-15

Fennema D, Phillips IR, Shephard EA. Trimethylamine and Trimethylamine N-Oxide, a Flavin-Containing Monooxygenase 3 (FMO3)-Mediated Host-Microbiome Metabolic Axis Implicated in Health and Disease [published correction appears in Drug Metab Dispos. 2016 Dec;44(12):1949]. Drug Metab Dispos. 2016;44(11):1839-1850. doi:10.1124/dmd.116.070615

Koh KK, Park SM, Quon MJ. Leptin and cardiovascular disease: response to therapeutic interventions. Circulation. 2008;117(25):3238-3249. doi:10.1161/CIRCULATIONAHA.107.741645

Elisardo C. Vasquez, Thiago M. C. Pereira, Veronica A. Peotta, Marcelo P. Baldo, Manuel Campos-Toimil, "Probiotics as Beneficial Dietary Supplements to Prevent and Treat Cardiovascular Diseases: Uncovering Their Impact on Oxidative Stress",Oxidative Medicine and Cellular Longevity, vol. 2019, Article ID 3086270, 11 pages,2019. https://doi.org/10.1155/2019/3086270

Bouassida A, Zalleg D, Bouassida S, et al. Leptin, its implication in physical exercise and training: a short review. J Sports Sci Med. 2006;5(2):172-181. Published 2006 Jun 1.

Dunbar, R.I.M., Baron, Rebecca, Frangou, Anna, Pearce, Eiluned, van Leeuwen, Edwin J.C.,Stow, Julie, Partridge, Giselle, MacDonald, Ian, Barra, Vincent, and van Vug, Mark. Social laughter is correlated with an elevated pain threshold. *Proc Biol Sci.* 2012 Mar 22; 279(1731): 1161–1167.

Strean, William B. PhD. Laughter prescription. *Can Fam Physician.* 2009 Oct; 55(10): 965–967.

Zahra Moshtag, Ezzati, Jaleh, Nasiri, Navideh, Ghafouri, Raziyeh. Effect of Humor Therapy on Blood Pressure of Patients Undergoing Hemodialysis. December 2017.*Journal of Research in Medical and Dental Science* 5(6) DOI: 10.24896/jrmds.20175615

Miller M, Fry WF. The effect of mirthful laughter on the human cardiovascular system. *Med Hypotheses.* 2009;73(5):636-639. doi:10.1016/j.mehy.2009.02.044.

Ryu KH, Shin HS, Yang EY. Effects of Laughter Therapy on Immune Responses in Postpartum Women. *J Altern Complement Med.* 2015;21(12):781-788. doi:10.1089/acm.2015.0053.

Voelkle, M. *Psychology and Aging,* online, Sept. 5, 2011.

Wenner, Melinda. Smile! It Could Make You Happier. *Scientific American Mind* 20, 5, 14-15 (September 2009) doi:10.1038/scientificamericanmind0909-14.

Doward, Jamie. Happy people really do work harder. *The Guardian.* Jul 10, 2010.

Childs CE, Calder PC, Miles EA. Diet and Immune Function. Nutrients. 2019;11(8):1933. Published 2019 Aug 16. doi:10.3390/nu11081933

Myles IA. Fast food fever: reviewing the impacts of the Western diet on immunity. Nutr J. 2014;13:61. Published 2014 Jun 17. doi:10.1186/1475-2891-13-61

Conde-Sieira M, Gesto M, Batista S, et al. Influence of vegetable diets on physiological and immune responses to thermal stress in Senegalese sole (Solea senegalensis). PLoS One. 2018;13(3):e0194353. Published 2018 Mar 22. doi:10.1371/journal.pone.0194353

Puertollano MA, Puertollano E, Alvarez de Cienfuegos G, de Pablo Martínez MA. Aceite de oliva, sistema inmune e infección [Olive oil, immune system and infection]. Nutr Hosp. 2010 Jan-Feb;25(1):1-8. Spanish. PMID: 20204249.

Liu P, Kerr BJ, Weber TE, Chen C, Johnston LJ, Shurson GC. Influence of thermally oxidized vegetable oils and animal fats on intestinal barrier function and immune variables in young pigs. J Anim Sci. 2014 Jul;92(7):2971-9. doi: 10.2527/jas.2012-5710. Epub 2014 May 30. PMID: 24879760.

Nieman DC, Henson DA, Austin MD, Sha W. Upper respiratory tract infection is reduced in physically fit and active adults. Br J Sports Med. 2011 Sep;45(12):987-92. doi: 10.1136/bjsm.2010.077875. Epub 2010 Nov 1. PMID: 21041243.

Martin SA, Pence BD, Woods JA. Exercise and respiratory tract viral infections. Exerc Sport Sci Rev. 2009;37(4):157-164. doi:10.1097/JES.0b013e3181b7b57b

Huang Z, Rose AH, Hoffmann PR. The role of selenium in inflammation and immunity: from molecular mechanisms to therapeutic opportunities. Antioxid Redox Signal. 2012;16(7):705-743. doi:10.1089/ars.2011.4145

Morey JN, Boggero IA, Scott AB, Segerstrom SC. Current Directions in Stress and Human Immune Function. Curr Opin Psychol. 2015;5:13-17. doi:10.1016/j.copsyc.2015.03.007

Sarkar D, Jung MK, Wang HJ. Alcohol and the Immune System. Alcohol Res. 2015;37(2):153-155.

Besedovsky L, Lange T, Born J. Sleep and immune function. Pflugers Arch. 2012;463(1):121-137. doi:10.1007/s00424-011-1044-0

Bennett MP, Lengacher C. Humor and Laughter May Influence Health IV. Humor and Immune Function. Evid Based Complement Alternat Med. 2009;6(2):159-164. doi:10.1093/ecam/nem149

Liu H, Waite LJ, Shen S, Wang DH. Is Sex Good for Your Health? A National Study on Partnered Sexuality and Cardiovascular Risk among Older Men and Women. J Health Soc Behav. 2016;57(3):276-296. doi:10.1177/0022146516661597

Murray DR, Haselton MG, Fales M, Cole SW. Falling in love is associated with immune system gene regulation. Psychoneuroendocrinology. 2019;100:120-126. doi:10.1016/j.psyneuen.2018.09.043

Book & Graphic design by Sarina Chang

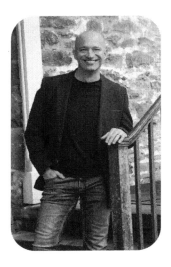

Photo by Drew Geraci

LARRY ROGOWSKY

Keep up with UBF on our social media!

Larry Rogowsky is known as Broadway's Health Coach. His practice as a Certified Nutrition Coach and Licensed Massage Therapist has served the wider theatrical community for decades, and has grown into a coaching practice for athletes, dancers, and high performers. Larry is passionate about wellness and helping individuals discover their most vibrant selves. Larry's work has led him to conduct seminars across North America on Effective Health and Lifestyle Practices. Larry couples his life in wellness along with a life in the arts. He is a Tony Award-winning Broadway Producer, with affiliations in Broadway shows including *Angels in America*, *Moulin Rouge!*, *Company*, and *Jagged Little Pill*. Larry is a father and husband.

Larry founded Urban Body Fix in 2001. With a passion for wellness and an engaging spirit, Larry has built a team of health professionals advocating for positive change and powerful choices in health and in life, for clients as well as medical practices.

For the individual, Urban Body Fix implements customizable health solutions that assist clients with overweight, fatigue, aching joints and more. For the health professional, Urban Body Fix's team enhances wellness services within a practice to increase productivity and effective communication, offering prevention-based solutions for superior health and happiness.